Pavlina Aleksova

Classification Of Pulp Stones

Pavlina Aleksova

Classification Of Pulp Stones

Detection method for Early detecting of Calculi In Other Organs

LAP LAMBERT Academic Publishing

Impressum / Imprint
Bibliografische Information der Deutschen Nationalbibliothek: Die Deutsche Nationalbibliothek verzeichnet diese Publikation in der Deutschen Nationalbibliografie; detaillierte bibliografische Daten sind im Internet über http://dnb.d-nb.de abrufbar.
Alle in diesem Buch genannten Marken und Produktnamen unterliegen warenzeichen-, marken- oder patentrechtlichem Schutz bzw. sind Warenzeichen oder eingetragene Warenzeichen der jeweiligen Inhaber. Die Wiedergabe von Marken, Produktnamen, Gebrauchsnamen, Handelsnamen, Warenbezeichnungen u.s.w. in diesem Werk berechtigt auch ohne besondere Kennzeichnung nicht zu der Annahme, dass solche Namen im Sinne der Warenzeichen- und Markenschutzgesetzgebung als frei zu betrachten wären und daher von jedermann benutzt werden dürften.

Bibliographic information published by the Deutsche Nationalbibliothek: The Deutsche Nationalbibliothek lists this publication in the Deutsche Nationalbibliografie; detailed bibliographic data are available in the Internet at http://dnb.d-nb.de.
Any brand names and product names mentioned in this book are subject to trademark, brand or patent protection and are trademarks or registered trademarks of their respective holders. The use of brand names, product names, common names, trade names, product descriptions etc. even without a particular marking in this work is in no way to be construed to mean that such names may be regarded as unrestricted in respect of trademark and brand protection legislation and could thus be used by anyone.

Coverbild / Cover image: www.ingimage.com

Verlag / Publisher:
LAP LAMBERT Academic Publishing
ist ein Imprint der / is a trademark of
OmniScriptum GmbH & Co. KG
Heinrich-Böcking-Str. 6-8, 66121 Saarbrücken, Deutschland / Germany
Email: info@lap-publishing.com

Herstellung: siehe letzte Seite /
Printed at: see last page
ISBN: 978-3-659-78324-1

Classification Of Pulp Stones

Detection method for Early detecting of Calculi In Other Organs

Pavlina Aleksova

2015

This book is mainly intended for doctors of stomatology and doctors with a specialization in endodontics. Residents of all stomatology areas and students of postgraduate (master), doctoral and postdoctoral studies should have this book in mind while preparing their possible themes of thesis. At the same time the undergraduate students who want to expand their knowledge of dental calcification and its connection with the entire pathologic calcification in the organism could find useful data in this monograph.

The practitioners of general medicine and the specialists of nephrology, gastroenterology, cardiology and all other specialties that meet pathologic calcification, in this book shall find answers for the patients with pathologic calcification. Physicians who have patients with associate unexplainable long-term headache could refer them to a doctor of stomatology for diagnosis and therapy of possible pulp stone pathology.

CONTENTS

Preface

The actual genesis of the dental calcification was the reason to make a wider research, meanwhile taking into consideration the endogenous disorders in the organism of similar nature.

Some data shows that most of the organs are surgically removed due to inadequate and correct diagnosis of the pathological calcification, than from affected organ.

Pulp stone, though of an unclear etiology, is clinically common. It potentially poses procedural difficulty to the endodontist and may also be a marker of an underlying systemic condition.

The large group of investigations in the world showed that the pathological calcification in soft and hard tissues in the organism is the most frequent chronic disease in humans. The characteristics of the disease, the incidence of new registered cases, the frequency of patients with recidive calculosis, the disease period length and the consecutive organ and organism repercussions, include the pathologic calcification in the group of illnesses with strong social impact.

Pulp stones or denticles are frequently found in the dental pulp. Regardless of the obvious endodontic problem of inhibiting access to the canals and their further treatment, they have not been given great importance. The latest experiences of scientific and practical research, including examinations of dental calcifications and their association with calcifications/calculi in the organism, have not been included in the literature.

The book contains personal experiences, one's own researches, views and results, specially the plan of diagnostics and associated with the pathologic calcification in organism.

A review of the literature was therefore performed, initially using the PubMed database and beginning the search with "pulp calcifications" and "pulp stones".

Contemporary textbooks in endodontology were also consulted, and an historic perspective gained from a number of older books and references.

At the end, the author thanks all those, which will find this book as necessity.

Author

Pavlina Aleksova

Skopje, 2015

Summary

Dental calcifications, known as denticles, are mineral deposits in the pulp tissue. They are discrete calcification bodies with definite, but very different localization, prevalence and histology.

The above-mentioned reasons led to establishing the target objectives of this project, as follows: to determine the morphological (according to the size, the shape, numeral prevalence, the localization) and structural features of dental calcifications, with new classification according to the structure. In addition, the aim of the project is to present new classification of dental pulp calcifications according to their composition with clinical implication, which results with connecting the dental and the pathologic calcification in the organism.

In the part of one's results, the standard histological analysis of the pulp tissues was being made on material provided from 240 endodontic ally extirpated dental pulps and 60 vertical cross-sections made after indicated tooth extractions.

Morphological features of dental calcifications show a wide range of variations. Regarding the structure of calcifications, 3 morphological images were identified: (1) Calcifications with morphological features similar to the structure of dentin, (2) Calcifications with lamellar concentric structure, and (3) Calcifications with granulated fine granular structure. According to the composition, the dental pulp stones can be classified as dentinal and non-dentinal.

Using the experience from present classifications of dental calcifications and the classifications of other diseases and syndromes, together with these results, can be a reason to propose a new classification of dental calcifications, according to the structure, new classification of dental calcifications, according to their composition. This can be confirmed histologically. The new classification will enable us to determinate the composition of denticles according to the age of patients, without any histological analysis.

When they are classified as non-dentinal, the dental practitioner is obligated to send the patient to subsequent or supplementary inspection, primarily ultrasonography survey first to abdomen, for early detecting of calcifications and calculus in other organs.

Kay words: pulp stones, pathological calcifications, classification, detection method, early detecting, calculi, other organs, practitioners, general medicine, nephrologists, gastroenterologists, cardiologists.

Introduction

Calcifications in the dental pulp, as a phenomenon with diverse occurrence and manifestation, represent a subject of constant interest not only from the perspective of being a separate dental entity but also because of the fact that they are interesting to observe and deal with from diagnostic and therapeutic aspect.

The fact that they are referred to as being provocateurs of pain with different intensity makes them cause difficulties in diagnosing.

When observed from therapeutic aspect, they appear to be of greater importance because they can make the access to the dental roots difficult or in some cases completely impossible, and they can also be the reason for groundless extraction of a tooth or a group of teeth.

Dental pulp calcifications are sometimes routine findings in oral radiographs and may later serve as an important diagnostic criterion for a hidden aspect of systemic illness.

The older clinical view is that pulp stones have no significance other than possibly causing difficulties during endodontic therapy, such as hindering canal location and negotiation.

1. Biological (syn. phisiological, standard, or normal) calcification

The current picture of the process of biological calcifications portrays the cells within the calcifying tissues as central factors controlling the deposition of mineral crystals in the extracellular matrix. The cell responds to hormones and second messengers, and other changes in its environment, regulating the concentration of ions within the extracellular matrix and secreting macromolecules whose properties determine the ability of the matrix to be calcified. The mitochondria within the cells accumulate calcium and phosphate, releasing these ions into the matrix as calcification progresses. Extracellular matrix vesicles, derived from the cells of some, but not all, calcifying matrices, provide sites for initial mineral deposition in many tissues. Among the macromolecules secreted by the cell, collagen provides the support for the hydroxyapatite crystals; proteoglycans serve to control the extent and/or progress of mineralization. The proteoglycans, glycoproteins, enzymes and the collagen itself, along with the cells, determine the nature of the matrix, while phosphoprotein, proteolipids, and phospholipids may serve as hydroxyapatite nucleators or as surfaces upon which apatite is deposited. But it is the interaction of many or all of these factors that determines the process of biological calcification and controls the properties of the calcified matrices [1].

Observations portray calcification processes as similar whether occurring normally or pathologically. Most forms of calcification are initiated by membranous organelles, i.e. extracellular, calcifying "matrix vesicles" or intracellular mitochondria. Matrix vesicles promote calcification through calcium-binding phospholipids and phosphatase activity. Mitochondria use a forceful, inwardly directed Ca and phosphate transport mechanism. After mineral initiation, the proliferation of mineral crystals is dependent on regulatory factors, such as extracellular $Ca2+$ and $PO4(3-)$ and other mineral inhibitors and promoters. Calcific diseases are defined as those in which (1) Ca uptake is early, (2) calcification is importantly related to dysfunction, and (3) the control of calcification may lead to decreased morbidity or enhanced diagnostic capability. Calcific diseases include such well-known entities as crystal deposition arthritis, atherosclerosis, calcific valvular sclerosis, tumor calcification, dental plaque, and dysfunctional calcification occurring in implanted cardiovascular devices [2].

In 2006, Garimella R, Bi X, Anderson HC, Camacho NP. with Fourier transform infrared imaging spectroscopy (FT-IRIS), characterize the mineral phase generated during MV-mediated in vitro mineralization.

Membrane-bound extracellular matrix vesicles play an important role in the de novo initiation and propagation of calcium-phosphate mineral formation in calcifying cartilage, bone, dentin, and in pathologic calcification. Characterization of the phase, composition, crystal size, and perfection provides valuable insight into the mechanism of the mineral deposition. Low concentrations of pyrophosphate (PPi) (< or = 0.01 mM) showed apatitic mineral while high concentrations showed immature calcium pyrophosphate dihydrate (CPPD) [3].

Matrix vesicles are extracellular 100-nanometer-diameter membrane-invested particles selectively located within the matrix of bone, cartilage, and predentin. They serve as the initial site of calcification in all skeletal tissues. Matrix vesicle biogenesis occurs by polarized budding and pinching off of vesicles from specific regions of the outer plasma membrane of chondrocytes, osteoblasts, and odontoblasts. Seeding of selected areas of matrix with matrix vesicles explains the localized distribution of subsequent zones of mineralization. Matrix vesicle biogenesis in the growth plate is linked to the chondrocyte cell cycle and reflects a stage in programmed cell death (apoptosis). Generation of initial hydroxyapatite mineral crystals occurs within the matrix vesicle membrane during Phase 1 of biologic mineralization. Phase 1 is controlled by phosphatases (including alkaline phosphatase) and Ca-binding molecules with which the matrix vesicles are well endowed. Phase 2 of biologic mineralization begins with breakdown of matrix vesicle membranes, exposing preformed hydroxyapatite to the extracellular fluid after which mineral crystal proliferation is governed by extracellular conditions. Phase 1 and Phase 2 of mineralization are under cellular control. Phase 1 is initiated by cells generating calcifiable matrix vesicles and releasing them into sites of intended calcification. Phase 2 is controlled by cells regulating extracellular ionic conditions and matrix composition [4].

Pathological (syn. abnormal) calcification

Pathological calcification usually is initiated by the biologic membranes of mitochondria or matrix vesicles. Mitochondria frequently initiate intracellular calcification. Matrix vesicles, derived from the outer membrane of cells by budding or cell disruption, initiate extracellular calcification in calcific tendonitis, apatite-deposition osteoarthritis, atherosclerosis, cardiac valvular calcification, tympanosclerosis, and other calcific diseases. Matrix vesicles and mitochondria usually initiate calcification through the interaction of phosphatase enzymes with calcium-binding phospholipids, both of which are membrane-bound. Hydroxyapatite (HA) crystals are formed first within the protective microenvironment of the membrane-enclosed microspace. Once formed and exposed to the extracellular fluid, HA crystals can serve as nuclei or templates, thus supporting progressive, autocatalytic mineral crystal proliferation [5].

Mineral-matrix interactions regulate the process of hydroxyapatite formation in bones and teeth. In mineralizing tissues, many anionic macromolecules bind to mineral. By means of this binding, such molecules are able to regulate the size and shape of the mineral crystals, determine the site of initial crystal deposition, and determine the type of mineral crystals deposited. Collagen, which provides a template for hydroxyapatite deposition; extracellular matrix vesicles, which provide a protected environment for crystal deposition; and noncollagenous matrix proteins that have high affinities for hydroxyapatite have all been shown to affect mineralization in vitro. Some of the noncollagenous proteins have been shown to be capable of promoting and inhibiting mineral formation and growth, depending on their concentration and whether they are immobilized or free in solution [6].

It is widely accepted that cells play a crucial role in the mineralization of dentin, cartilage and bone. The initial locus of calcification appears to be the matrix vesicle, a 200 nm submicroscopic extracellular, membrane-invested particle which is shed from the osteoblast, chondrocyte, or odontoblast and carries into the matrix calcifiable lipids and phosphatases. During Phase 1 of mineralization, the initiation phase, apatite appears within matrix vesicles, probably preceded by amorphous calcium phosphate. Initially, acidic phospholipids of matrix vesicles may attract calcium to form complexes with phosphate and protein. In vitro studies of cartilage slices and isolated matrix vesicles indicate the essentiality of vesicle phosphatases for mineral initiation. In pathological calcification is self-sustaining. Given physiological amounts of $Ca2+$ and $PO43(-)$, calcification will spread by crystal proliferation into the extracellular matrix surrounding vesicles (Phase 2). During Phase 2 the rate of crystal proliferation is controlled by matrical factors: Collagen can orient and apparently promote apatite formation. Proteoglycans, pyrophosphate, gamma-carboxyglutamic acid-containing proteins and phosphoproteins in calcifying matrix bind $Ca2+$ by their anionic subgroups, and all have been shown to impede hydroxyapatite formation in vitro. The latter substances are visualized as regulating Phase 2 by inhibiting mineral growth. The calcification process involves an interaction of all of the above. When viewed as a 2-phase phenomenon, it is possible to integrate each of these factors into a comprehensive concept of biological mineralization [7].

Boskey AL., Boyan BD., Schwartz Z. in 1997 confirm that extracellular matrix vesicles (MVs) are associated with initial calcification in a variety of tissues, but the mechanisms by which they promote mineralization are not certain [8].

Calcification is a rock-hard mix of the most plentiful minerals in the body: calcium and phosphorus. Normally this calcium phosphate mix is essential for building bones and teeth. But as we age, and sometimes when we are still young, some of it goes haywire, stiffening arteries, roughing up skin, destroying teeth, blocking kidneys.

Calcification doubles in the body about every three or four years. We can have it as teenagers and not notice, although it mysteriously accelerates in some athletes. Then as we age and also live longer, it becomes so endemic that most people over seventy have it. As we learn more about it, calcification is competing to be the leading medical disorder: dental pulp stones, hardening of the arteries, kidney stones, pitcher's elbow, bone spurs [9].

In normal healthy individuals, mineral formation is restricted to specialized tissues which form the skeleton and the dentition. Within these tissues, mineral formation is tightly controlled both in growth and development and in normal adult life. The mechanism of calcification in skeletal and dental tissues has been under investigation for a considerable period. One feature common to almost all of these normal mineralization mechanisms is the elaboration of matrix vesicles, small (20–200 nm) membrane particles, which bud off from the plasma membrane of mineralizing cells and are released into the pre-mineralized organic matrix. The first crystals which form on this organic matrix are seen in and around matrix vesicles. Pathologic ectopic mineralization is seen in a number of human genetic and acquired diseases, including calcification of joint cartilage resulting in osteoarthritis and mineralization of the cardiovasculature resulting in exacerbation of atherosclerosis and blockage of blood vessels. Surprisingly, increasing evidence supports the contention that the mechanisms of soft tissue calcification are similar to those seen in normal skeletal development. In particular, matrix vesicle-like membranes are observed in a number of ectopic calcifications [10].

Biomineralization

Biomineralization is a highly regulated process that plays a major role during the development of skeletal tissues. Despite its obvious importance, little is known about its regulation. Previously, it has been demonstrated that retinoic acid (RA) stimulates terminal differentiation and mineralization of growth plate chondrocytes (Iwamoto, M., I.M. Shapiro, K. Yagumi, A.L. Boskey, P.S. Leboy, S.L. Adams, and M. Pacifici. 1993. Exp. Cell Res. 207:413-420). Wang W. and Kirsch T., evidence that RA treatment of growth plate chondrocytes caused a series of events eventually leading to mineralization of these cultures: increase in cytosolic calcium concentration, followed by up-regulation of annexin II, V, and VI gene expression, and release of annexin II-, V-, VI- and alkaline phosphatase-containing matrix vesicles. Cotreatment of growth plate chondrocytes with RA and BAPTA-AM, a cell permeable Ca2+ chelator, inhibited the up-regulation of annexin gene expression and mineralization of these cultures. Interestingly, only matrix vesicles isolated from RA-treated cells that contained annexins, were able to take up Ca2+ and mineralize, whereas vesicles isolated from untreated or RA/BAPTA-treated cells, that contained no or only little annexins were not able to take up Ca2+ and mineralize. Cotreatment of chondrocytes with RA and EDTA revealed that increases in the cytosolic calcium concentration were due to influx of extracellular calcium. Interestingly, the novel 1,4-benzothiazepine derivative K-201, a specific annexin Ca2+ channel blocker, or antibodies specific for annexin II, V, or VI inhibited the increases in cytosolic calcium concentration in RA-treated chondrocytes. These findings indicate that annexins II, V, and VI form Ca2+ channels in the plasma membrane of terminally differentiated growth plate chondrocytes and mediate Ca2+ influx into these cells. The resulting increased cytosolic calcium concentration leads to a further up-regulation of annexin II, V, and VI gene expression, the release of annexin II-, V-, VI- and alkaline phosphatase-containing matrix vesicles, and the initiation of mineralization by these vesicles [11].

MVs facilitate mineralization by providing enzymes that modify inhibitory factors in the extracellular matrix, as well as by providing a protected environment in which mineral ions can accumulate. Bone and tooth mineralization is critically regulated by mineralization inhibitors [12].

Calcifications in the dental pulp, as a phenomenon with diverse prevalence and manifestation, represent a subject of constant interest not only from the perspective of being a separate dental entity but also because of the fact that they are interesting to observe and deal with from diagnostic and therapeutic aspect. The fact that they are referred to as being provocateurs of pain with different intensity makes them cause difficulties in diagnosing.

2. Terminology of dental calcifications

These bodies under the term of "dental pulp nodules" were first mentioned by Norman and Johnston in 1921. This term has in time been replaced by the term "pulp stones", "denticles", "dental calcifications" or as "calcified deposits". In recent literature the term "dental nodules" has appeared. Regardless of the historical transformation in their nomination, they have been des-cribbed as unique calcifying changes including "diffuse pulp calcification", i.e. "dystrophic calcification".

3. Etiology of dental calcifications

Despite several microscopic and histochemical studies, the exact cause of such pulp calcifications remains largely unknown. However, a number of conditions have been possible causative factors such as: caries, deep fillings, and chronic inflammation, [13,14], operative procedures, periodontal diseases, epithelial rests in the pulp tissue, orthodontic tooth movement, [15,16], degeneration, inductive interactions between the epithelium and pulp tissue [17], age [18], circulatory disturbances in pulp tissue [19], idiopathic factors, genetic predisposition [20], fluoride supplementation [21], Marfan syndrome [22], nanobacteria/ CNPs [23,24].

Nanobacteria can be found in part of the dental calcifications, dental plaque, and blood, calcifications of other organs and in serum. They cause the formation of calcifications [25,26]. They are cytotoxic, sterile – filterable, gram-negative, atypical bacteria discovered in the blood of mammals [25].

In calcification, all that is needed for crystal formation to start is nidi (nuclei) and an environment of available dissolved components at or near saturation concentrations, along with the absence of inhibitors for crystal formation. Calcifying nanoparticles (CNP) are the first calcium phosphate mineral containing particles isolated from human blood and were detected in numerous pathologic calcification related diseases.

Controversy and critical role of CNP as nidi and triggering factor in human pathologic calcification are discussed [27].

The mineral phase of many kinds of hard tissue in organisms is called biologic apatite (BA). Pure hydroxyapatite (HA) has the formula $Ca_{10}(PO_4)_6(OH)_2$. BA additionally contains several other ions, mainly carbonate but also trace amounts of other anions such as HPO_4^{2-}, Cl^-, and F^-. Other cation elements are also present in minor amounts including Mg^{2+}, Na^+, and Fe^{2+}. BA is the primary mineral of normal bone and teeth [28].

By definition, pathologic calcification refers to the deposition of calcium phosphates (CaP) or other calcific salts at sites, which would not normally have become mineralized. Abnormal accumulation can occur in areas of tissue damage (dystrophic calcification), in hypercalcemic or hyper parathyroid states [29].

Kidney and bladder stones, dental pulp stones, some gall stones, salivary gland stones and many others are the most common diseases involving extra skeletal calcification [30,31].

Most pathologic calcifications throughout the body contain mixtures of carbonate-substituted HA and octacalcium phosphate. According to the Merck Manuel, these ultramicroscopic crystals occur in snowball-like clumps. Those clumps can cause severe inflammation [32].

Structures similar to these nanometer-sized snowballs were discovered almost two decades ago in blood and blood products [33]. These structures, called calcifying nanoparticles (CNP), were detected in numerous pathologic calcification related diseases [34–37]. CNP are the first CaP mineral containing particles isolated from human blood.

Chemical analysis using energy-dispersive x-ray microanalysis (EDX) of these mineral layers shows Ca and P peaks [38-41].

Dentin dysplasia (DD), a rare anomaly is an autosomal dominant hereditary disturbance in dentin formation affecting either the primary or both the dentitions in approximately one patient in every 100,000 [42]. It was Ballschmiede [43] in 1920 who first reported such a condition as 'rootless teeth' and in 1939 Rushton termed this condition as DD [44]. On the basis of radiological findings, Witkop in 1972 classified DD into type I: Radicular DD and type II: Coronal dentin dysplasia [45], report Sangamesh G. Fulari and Deepti P. Tambake [46].

While the gross morphology of pulp stones has been described and is well documented the irregular, diffuse calcifications cannot be adequately characterized microscopically because of the lack of specific structural detail, and consequently most authors have regarded them as "amorphous mineral deposits" [Brabant et al., 1953; Stanley, 1965; Taatz and Widmaier, 1962; Sicher, 1966 and others]. Whereas in pulp stones a definite organic matrix is the site of apatite nucleation (similar to dentine, bone, or cartilage), inform Plačková A. and Vahl J. in 1974 year [47].

4. Classifications of dental calcifications, pulp stones, denticles

While the gross morphology of pulp stones has been described and is well documented the irregular, diffuse calcifications cannot be adequately characterized microscopically because of the lack of specific structural detail, and consequently most authors have regarded them as "amorphous mineral deposits" [Brabant et al., 1953; Stanley, 1965; Taatz and Widmaier, 1962; Sicher, 1966 and others]. Whereas in pulp stones a definite organic matrix is the site of apatite nucleation (similar to dentine, bone, or cartilage), inform Plačková A. and Vahl J. in 1974 year [47].

Table 1. Classifications of dental calcifications

Classification	Year	Investigator	Titles
Embedded, adherent and free	1956	Johnson & Bevelander	Histogenesis and Pulpal calcification
Laminated and without distinct laminations	1973	Appleton & Williams	Ultrastructural observations on the calcification of human dental pulp
True and false and diffuse or amorphous	1973	Mjör and Pindborg	Histology of the human tooth
True and false (orthodentine and fibrodentine)	1983	Moss-Salentijn & Klyvert	Epithelially induced denticles in the pulps of recently erupted, noncarious human premolars
Fibrodentine (laminated pattern) and orthodentine	1988	Moss-Salentijn & Klyvert	Calcified structures in human dental pulps
Round or ovoid and assume no particular shape	2006	Pashley & Liewehr	Structure and Functions of the Dentin-Pulp Complex

Pulp stones are discrete calcifications and are amongst changes that include more diffuse pulp calcifications such as dystrophic calcification. Stones may exist freely within the pulp tissue or be attached to or embedded in dentine [48].

Two types of calcified bodies in the dental pulp have been described Moss-Salentijn & Klyvert 1983: denticles possessing a central cavity filled with epithelial remnants surrounded peripherally by odontoblasts, and pulp stones being compact degenerative masses of calcified tissues [49].

The calcifications in dental pulp appeared to consist of discrete, smooth-surfaced laminated denticles and irregularly shaped, non-laminated denticles, together with a diffuse calcification characterized by small foci scattered throughout the fibrous pulp matrix.

Both the laminated and non-laminated denticles had an organic matrix consisting of collagen fibres together with a background of electron dense material between the fibres [50].

The composition of the calcified bodies varies. They may be composed of "ortho" dentin, no tubular "fibro" dentin or irregular calcified material. Frequently the calcified bodies are conglomerates of these different tissues. The traditional classification of true and false denticles, based on histological characteristics, is difficult to maintain in view of this complexity of composition. [51].

Prof. Irvin Glickman B.S. in the 1954 year, the degree of degenerative pulps changes is related to the severity of the systemic disturbance [52]. Pulp calcifications occurring throughout the dentition are uncommon and are usually associated with systemic or genetic disorders of dentine [53].

Pulp stones have been reported in patients with systemic or genetic diseases such as van der Woude syndrome [54].

Case reports exist where (generalized) pulp stones are found in the dentitions of individuals with various conditions. These include tumoral calcinosis (Burkes et al. 1991), dentine dysplasia type II (Diamond 1989, Dean et al. 1997), Saethre-Chotzen syndrome (Goho 1998), elfin faces syndrome (Kelly & Barr 1975), familial expansive osteolysis (Mitchell et al. 1990), Ehlers Danlos syndrome type I (Hollister 1978, Pope et al. 1992), osteogenesis imperfecta type I (Lukinmaa et al. 1987, Levin et al. 1988) and otodental syndrome (Sedano et al. 2001). Unusual cases of idiopathic generalized pulp stone formation have been reported (Weiss 1927, Hitchin 1936, Siskos & Georgopoulou 1990), although sometimes a genetic predisposition has been noted (Rao et al. 1970, VanDenBerghe et al. 1999), [51].

Structurally, there are true and false pulp stones; the distinction being morphological. A third type, 'diffuse' or 'amorphous' pulp stones, is more irregular in shape than false pulp stones, occurring in close association with blood vessels [55]. True pulp stones are made of dentine and lined by odontoblasts, whereas false pulp stones are formed from degenerating cells of the pulp that mineralize. Such mineralization occurs in stages; initially cell nests become enclosed by concentrically arranged fibres (i.e. an organic phase precedes mineralization) which then become impregnated with mineral salts. Calcified increments are then added [48]. Based on location, pulp stones can be embedded, adherent and free. Embedded stones are formed in the pulp but with ongoing physiological dentine formation they become enclosed (sometimes fully) within the canal walls (Philippas 1961). They are found most frequently in the apical portion of the root, and the presence of odontoblasts and calcified tissue resembling dentine can occur on the peripheral aspect of these stones [48]. Adherent pulp stones are simply less attached to dentine than embedded pulp stones; the difference between adherent and embedded can be subjective, but adherent stones are never fully enclosed by dentine. Adherent and embedded pulp stones can interfere with root canal treatment if they cause significant occlusion of canals or are located at a curve. They may also become dislodged. Free pulp stones are found within the pulp tissue proper and are the most commonly seen type on radiographs.

Stones can be further subdivided into those with distinct concentric laminations and those without distinct laminations. Laminated pulp stones are not usually associated with smaller pulp stones, whereas non laminated stones are rougher and may have smaller stones attached to their surfaces [50].

Calcifications of pulp traditionally, calcified bodies in the dental pulp have been classified on the basis of their structural characteristics. The classification by Kronfield is most commonly used [49]. 1. "true" denticles (composed of tubular-ortho dentin), 2. "false" denticles (composed of concentric layers of calcified material not resembling dentin), 3. "diffuse calcifications" (small calcified deposits scattered throughout the pulp tissue). Firstly, one may easily, but incorrectly, assume that the histological properties of these calcified bodies are related to their mode of development (i.e. true denticles develop as the result of epithelio-mesenchymal interactions, while false denticles form on a calcified nidus). As shown below, such a strict relationship does not exist. Secondly, most pulpal calcifications are conglomerates of different tissues: orthodentin, regular, and irregular calcified material, so that a strict classification becomes nearly impossible [56-58].

Orthodentin, tubular dentin, may be detected both in denticles and in pulp stones. Denticles, formed as the result of epithelio-mesenchymal interactions, are composed of tubular dentin in the earliest stage of their development [16,17]. Odontoblasts line the periphery of the denticles, but as the diameters of these calcified bodies increase, most or all of the odontoblasts become reduced in height and apparently perish [59]. The lumina of their dentinal tubules undergo sclerosis and are no longer evident light microscopically [17]. Pulp stones are developed initially as an amorphous calcified nidus, but they may acquire peripheral masses of orthodentin (complete with predentin border and odontoblasts) as they increase in dimension [48,56,60]. It has been suggested that all dental papilla cells initially undergo an induction by odontogenic epithelium and that for a limited period of time they remain capable of responding to an appropriate challenge--such as the presence of a pulp stone--by differentiating into odontoblasts and producing dentin [60]. Thus, the presence of "true dentin" might not necessarily be an indication of direct epithelio-mesenchymal interactions, although it frequently is. It could equally be an indication that healthy young pulp tissue has responded to an appropriate stimulus. Regular calcified material may be found in the peripheral. Pulp stones increase in size by gradual deposition of layers of regular calcified material on the surface of the irregular calcified nidal core. The most striking feature of the resulting calcified body is that it appears laminated light microscopically. A laminated pulp stone is composed of layers of concentrically arranged collagen fibers and electron-dense interfibrillar material into which hydroxyapatite mineral has been deposited [61,62]. The regular structure of this material as well as the presence of an uncalcified peripheral border which gradually becomes calcified suggest that it has been deposited by some kind of hard tissue-forming cell. However, thus far such cells have not been identified. The tissue has been described as non tubular fibro dentin ("osteodentin'). It resembles dentin formed in older teeth, particularly dentin found near the root apex. Similar layers of non tubular fibro dentin are also frequently found on the surface of any denticle that remains free in the pulp tissue rather than becoming attached or embedded, as is more usual. Thus, the deposition of regular layers of non tubular fibro dentin may just reflect the particular ability of a somewhat older pulp tissue to respond to the challenge which the presence of a pulp stone or denticle represents. Irregular calcified material may be found at the core of most pulp stones but also occasionally on the surface of a laminated pulp stone or even on the surface of a denticle. Diffuse calcifications are composed entirely of this material. Irregular calcified deposits consist of an irregular matrix of collagen fibers and electron-dense inter fibrillar material into which hydroxyapatite crystallites have been deposited. The collagen fibers appear to be part of the normal intercellular matrix of the pulp tissue. These calcified bodies, which may become quite large, have an irregular periphery. They grow by addition of mineral to adjacent matrix fibers [47,61,63]. Calcify Metamorphosis is defined as a pulpal response to trauma that is characterized by deposition of hard tissue within the root canal space and is commonly found in young adults in the anterior region of the mouth [56].

Pulp stone, though of an unclear etiology, is clinically common. It potentially poses procedural difficulty to the endodontist and may also be a marker of an underlying systemic condition [64].

R. Kronfeld and P. E. Boyle 1953 year, proposed that histologically classified into "true" or "false" forms, the former containing irregular dentine and the latter being degenerative pulp calcifications [65,66].

Johnson & Bevelander 1956, stones may exist freely within the pulp tissue or be attached to or embedded in dentine [48]. Based on location, pulp stones can be embedded, adherent and free. Embedded stones are formed in the pulp but with ongoing physiological dentine formation they become enclosed (sometimes fully) within the canal walls (Philippas 1961). They are found most frequently in the apical portion of the root, and the presence of odontoblasts and calcified tissue resembling dentine can occur on the peripheral aspect of these stones (Johnson & Bevelander 1956). Adherent pulp stones are simply less attached to dentine than embedded pulp stones; the difference between adherent and embedded can be subjective, but adherent stones are never fully enclosed by dentine. Adherent and embedded pulp stones can interfere with root canal treatment if they cause significant occlusion of canals or are located at a curve [51].

Two types of calcified bodies in the dental pulp have been described (Moss-Salentijn & Klyvert 1983): denticles possessing a central cavity filled with epithelial remnants surrounded peripherally by odontoblasts, and pulp stones being compact degenerative masses of calcified tissues [17].

Other studies have noted problems with the above classification and new histological classifications have been proposed [67,68].

Kronfield has classified pulp calcifications into discrete (denticles and pulp nodules) and diffuse types based on the morphology. Seltzer has classified pulp stones based on their structure into true and false types, and based on size into fine and diffuse mineralization, and based on location into embedded and free types. [69]

Calcific Metamorphosis Calcific metamorphosis is defined as a pulpal response to trauma that is characterized by deposition of hard tissue within the root canal space and is commonly found in young adults in the anterior region of the mouth [56].

According Bernice Thomas et al. [59], possible modes of development generally, two different modes of development of pulpal calcifications have been proposed: initial calcification of isolated pulp tissue components; and epithelio-mesenchymal interactions.

Calcification of tissue components many researchers considered only a single mechanism: the initial calcification of a component of pulp tissue (ground substance, necrotic cell remnants, collagen fibril), which is believed to serve as a nidus upon which calcified material is eventually deposited, either in a concentric lamellar or in a radial fashion [19,56]. Bab et al. and Appleton et al. have provided ultrastructural descriptions of this process [50,61], Several researchers' suggests that a substantial number of pulpal calcifications develops in similar manner, even in preeruptive teeth [17]. This mode of development is mostly involved in the formation of all of the calcified structures in the coronal pulp and all of the calcified structures that form either as part of normal age related changes or as the result of local pathological changes of the pulp tissue (coronal and radicular). In any connective tissue, various calcification promoters and inhibitors are present. Calcification may occur in a normally no calcifying tissue, such as the pulp, when the balance between the two is disturbed; for example, by the local breakdown of inhibitors (e.g. proteoglycan complexes). Sundell et al. have stated that vascular damage following trauma or a "local metabolic dysfunction" is the precipitating factor for the development of a nidus [19]. There exists a close spatial relationship between calcified structures and the blood vessels and/or nerves of the pulp [19, 60,70].

Occasionally these nidi (or foci) are located inside vascular lumina or in neurovascular bundles, mostly in the pulps of deciduous teeth during shedding. While in the latter the calcifications probably associated with the degeneration of the nerves themselves, in most other instances the observed close spatial relationship between calcifications and neurovascular bundles may be coincidental due to the richness of the neurovascular supply of the pulp [48], which makes it nearly impossible for the calcified structure not to be close to a neurovascular bundle. Certain investigators have suggested that pulpal calcifications may be associated with certain systemic conditions such as arteriosclerosis. In a radiographic study, Stafne et al. reported the incidence of calcifications in pulp chambers was correlated with the documented existence of some non dental systemic conditions [16]. While the incidence in normal individuals was 46%, it was somewhat, but not significantly, higher in patients with arteriosclerosis (53%), osteitis deforming (55.7%).

Epithelio-mesenchymal interactions this mode of development has been suggested for a second, much smaller group of calcified bodies in the dental pulp. Baume et al. [56], reported this theory of development suggests that epithelial strands are detached from the enamel organ during tooth development. Later, these strands become isolated in the dental papilla where they interact with the papilla mesenchyme, resulting in the physiologically normal differentiation of odontoblasts around the strands. Detached epithelial strands or cell nests have been observed in the papilla mesenchyme [71,72], and studies [16,17,71], have shown what can be interpreted to be developmental stages of the resulting calcified bodies. Typically, an epithelial strand is found at the core of each of these bodies during the initial stages of development. Odontoblasts deposit dentin as they move away from this epithelium. The resulting structures are initially hollow, not solid. They may be thimble-shaped, with their concavities facing apically, or approximately spherical, with a central cavity surrounded on all sides by dentin. Since, in addition, these structures are initially composed of true dentin; the use of the term denticles (small teeth) for them is most suited. These distinctively shaped denticles are found only in those locations where a root sheath is present or in the furcation areas of multirooted teeth where epithelial extensions subdivide the cervical opening of the enamel organ.

5. Materials and methods for obtaining one's results

The research was made on 240 endodontically extirpated dental pulps of teeth with endodontic diagnosis of chronic pulpitis and 60 vertical cross-sections made after indicated tooth extractions.

TABLE 2. Distribution of 240 endodontically extirpated dental pulps:

Side	Left								Right							
Tooth	8	7	6	5	4	3	2	1	1	2	3	4	5	6	7	8
Maxilla		10	20	20	4	2	1		1	2	10	10	10	20		
Mandible		20	20		2	10		2	2		10	10	10	30	4	

TABLE 3. Distribution of 60 dental pulps after vertical cross-sections made after indicated tooth extractions

Side	Left								Right							
Tooth	8	7	6	5	4	3	2	1	1	2	3	4	5	6	7	8
Maxilla		1	2	2	2	2	1	1	1	1	1		2	1		
Mandible	2	2	2	1		2	2	1	1	1	3	4	2			

TABLE 4. Distribution of endodontically extirpated dental pulps according age

The age	20-30	30-40	40-50	50-60	20-30	30-40	40-50	50-60
Dental pulps	55	90	45	50	++	+ + +	+	+

The standard histological analysis of the pulp tissue was being made on material provided by means of endodontic extirpations and vertical cross-section made after indicated teeth extractions. For the purpose of histological processing, various methods and procedures were used, such as:

• **Fixation**

Fixation is such important method in stabilization of the proteins and preservation of nucleus and cells structures, lead is with water solution of formaldehyde.

All tissues samples, were in 10% formalin, concerning 4% water solution of formaldehyde. The volume ratio of the formalin toward tissues material, bringing at least 10:1.

Short time of the fixation – 48 hours.

• **Decalcination**

Necessary for paraffin's tissues moulds, is to soften with the help of process of decalcination with the combination technique of tissue upper process of decalcination, with hurry and spore decalcination.

The rich decalcinate in procedure of the hurry decalcination - water solution of nitrogen acid, with composition:

Formalin	10 ml.
Water destilate	80 ml.
Nitrogen acid	10 ml.

In the procedure of spore and control decalcination: 3% water solution of nitrogen acid and 5% water solution of formic acid:

Decalcinat of nitrogenic acid:		Decalcinat of formic acid:	
Formalin	15 ml.	Formalin	15 ml.
Water distillate	82 ml.	Water distillate	80 ml.
Nitrogen acid	3 ml.	Formic acid	5 ml.

With method of hurry and spore decalcination – prepare materials of extracted teeth, in the time of 2 to 12 mounts. Dental pulps – method of spore control decalcination in the time of 30 min. to 150 min. The half of material from dental pulps – procedure of the postpone decalcination. The first obtain is standards tissues sections, next tissue sample is rehydration and return in decalcinate in the time for spore and control decalcination.

- **Tissue processing**

Tissue processing is realized in the tissue processor Citadela 2000 – Shandon – method of standard and shortened procedure.

Method of standard tissue processing:

	Fluid	Time/hour
1	10% formalin	1
2	70% alcohol	1
3	95% alcohol	1
4	100% alcohol	2
5	100% alcohol	2
6	100% alcohol	1
7	100% alcohol	1
8	100% alcohol/Xylol	1
9	Xylol	2
10	Xylol	2
11	paraffin	2
12	paraffin	2

Method of standard tissue processing:

Container	Fluid	Time/min.
1	10% formalin	5
2	70% alcohol	10
3	95% alcohol	10
4	100% alcohol	15
5	100% alcohol	15
6	100% alcohol	15
7	Xylol	20
8	Xylol	15
9	paraffin	15
10	paraffin	20

- **Provision of paraffin sections**

Paraffin sections itself with slide microtome "Leica" and "Reinchard".

The stoutness of the sections: 4 – 5 microns, with rightly of the blade longitudinal.

- **Standard staining**

Standard hematoxylin and eosin staining:

Hematoxylin: Gill*s III (Merck)

Eosin: Eosin Y (Merck)

Method:

	Procedure		Time/min.
	deparafinisation		
1	Xylol		2
2	Xylol		2
	rehydration		
3	alcohol	96%	2
4	alcohol	80%	2
5	alcohol	50%	2
6,7,8	water		3 x
9	hematoxylin		2-4
10	washing/water		3 x
11	lithium carbonate	1%	3 x
12	washing / water		3 x
13	eosin		2-4
14	washing / water		3 x
	dehydration		
15	alcohol	50%	2
16	alcohol	80%	2
17	alcohol	96%	2
18	alcohol	100%	2
19	alcohol	100%	2
	clearing		
20	Xylol		2
21	Xylol		2

• **Differential coloring**

Differential coloring: von Kossa and Giemsa

Coloring: von Kossa:

1%   water solution of silver nitrate

2,5% Sodium thiosulfate

1%   picrofuxin

Method:

1	leading of the sections in the distillation water
2	leading in the Na carbonate and expose of the strong light 10 – 60 min.
3	washing of the sections in the distillation water
4	treated with Sodium thiosulfate 5 min.
5	washing in the distillation water
6	different coloring
7	dehydration, purgation

Coloring - Giemsa (Merck):

Finish solution - Giemsa (Merck) in of vinegar acid to droughty

Method:

1	leading of the sections in the distillation water
2	leading in the distillation water of Ph 6.8
3	leading in solution Giemsa 1 hour.
4	washing in the distillation water
5	leading in 0,5% water solution of vinegar acid to red coloring
6	washing in the running water
7	droughty, dehydration, purgation

Coloring - Masson trichrom:

Finish solutions - Masson trichrom (Merck)

Method:

1	deparafinisation
2	application of solution A
3	washing in the distillation water
4	leading in solution B 5 min.
5	washing in the distillation water
6	leading in solution C 2 – 5 min.
7	washing in the running water
8	leading in 1% waters solution of vinegar acid 2 min.
9	droughty, dehydration, purgation

- **Microscopy and morphological analysis**

    Histological preparations – microscope Nikon Labophot 2

- **Photography**

    Laica with magnify from 10 x 4, 10 x 10, 10 x 20, 10 x 40 and 10 x 60.

- **Hardware and software** - Image analyzer Lucia M.

6. MORPHOLOGY OF RADICULAR DENTAL CALCIFICATIONS

6.1 The size of calcifications

Regarding the size, calcifications show a wide range of variations. The findings show values smaller than 1 micron, up to 1cm, measured per samples with continuous areas of calcifications which fill in almost the whole pulp, in a longitudinal direction. The transverse section is within the limits of 20 to 200 microns, whereas the longitudinal section is up to 500 microns.

6.2 The shape of calcifications

According to shape, 2 groups are identified.

1. The first group consists of calcifications of oval shape, which have a degree of bending similar to circle or spherical objects; these calcifications are nodular.
2. The second group of calcifications consists of calcifications which are of irregular shape, corner-like, except the bigger ones, which are relatively elongated.

6.3 Numeral prevalence

According to this morphological parameter, it results with distributions of wider borders.

The spherical calcifications show tendency of grouping according to their number with average value of 3 calcifications per volume of one pulp.

The irregular calcifications do not show tendency of grouping themselves according to their numerical occurrence per volume in one pulp, although at average they are more numerous in their occurrence from the spherical calcifications.

6.4 Localization of calcifications

Perceived in longitudinal direction, with ordinary segmentation of the pulp in 3 thirds, calcifications are localized in each third as well as in the transition areas among them. Spherical calcifications occur more often in the middle third, whereas irregular calcifications do not show any predilection.

Regarding the transverse measuring of the pulp, parts of spherical calcifications are closer to the lateral sides of the pulp i.e. to the surface of the pulp. Irregular calcifications are situated more centrally, as well as across the whole width of the pulp.

6.5 Structure of calcifications

Regarding the structure of calcifications, the analysis made according to the method of light microscopy by making use of standard differential histochemical coloring identified three morphological images:

I.   Calcifications with morphological features similar to the structure of dentin,

II.   Calcifications with lamellar concentric structure, and

III.   Calcifications small granular structure.

I.   Calcifications with morphological features similar to the structure of dentin
-   show greater affinity to eosin i.e. get colored in intense red, unlike the other two groups of calcifications, which further implies that there is a greater quantity of organic matrix in them.

Within the scope of visibility with the light microscopy there can be identified fine tubular-trabecular structures which with some changes get radial layout, and with other changes get anarchical layout.

The periphery of the spherules i.e. the periphery of the pulp calculi is colored more lightly in the middle area and creates a morphological image similar to crown, which is with different width and with longitudinally different radial projections to inwards and to outwards.

This part of the spherule is suitable to dentin with smaller quantity of calcium, the one being known as predentin.

The middle part of the spherules is more intensively amphophilic i.e. it has affinity to bond more hematoxylin and eosin.

This affinity for colors suggests greater presence of both organic matrix and greater quantity of calcium salts.

The analogy towards the normal structure of dentin and its morphogenesis during the formation implies that this zone is a zone of calcified mature dentin.

In some of the samples, on areas where sections were made, there were obtained junction zones of interconnection between the dentin mass of the spherule and the basic mass of the peripulped dentin, which represents another parameter that unambiguously shows that there is identical histogenesis of both the tooth dentine and these spherical more or less calcified structures.

II. Calcifications with lamellar concentric structure are spherical at shape

They are nodules similar in size as the previous ones. These calcifications get more intensively colored with hematoxylin i.e. they show more intensive basophilia unlike the denticles.

The depositing of calcium salts is rough with no presence of fine trabecular – tubular structures, visible as it is the case with the denticles. In search of associative morphological comparisons, the section of these calculi to a significant extent reminds of the tree circles.

The lamellarity and concentrity of the discolorations of the transverse sections of these calculi imply that there is organic smell, as initial nidus, with timely protracted circular, organically interpolated encrustment with calcium salts.

These morphological changes known as false denticles, fall under the wider group of dystrophic calcifications and as being such, from terminological perspective, they probably deserve to be referred to with another name.

III. Calcifications with granulated fine granular structure

In this group, according to their shape, fall calcifications with spherical oval shape and calcifications with irregular shape.

These two calcifications have pretty similar structure, with present zones of encrustments which are at their shape amorphous and uniformed, up to zones with fine granulated material.

Common for all the calcifications that belong to this group is the intensive coloring with hematoxylin i.e. the basophilic coloring which implies that there is the greatest presence of calcium salts in them when compared to the previous two groups.

The organic matrix is maximum reduced, so that after the decalcination phase it becomes transparent and in some places it appears to be missing; it is there where empty cracked and lacunar spaces are formed.

This type of uniformed calcification shows that there is a continuous time dynamics in the depositing of calcium, within a short time interval.

Post-necrotic changes, in the case of appropriately replaced homeostatic mechanisms, are precondition for the formation of this type of calcifications.

6.6 Composition of calcifications

The results obtained from the carried out examinations showed that dental calcifications can be classified as: dentinal and non-dentinal.

1. The dentinal calcifications are spherical, nodular, solitary and more numerous; they contain greater amount of organic matrix; they occur at early age and have hamartomatous aspect.

2. The non-dentinal calcifications could be nodular spherical, irregular in shape or with punctform encrustations. They contain smaller amount of organic matrix, they occur in the middle or older age and have inflammatory dystrophic background.

TABLE 4.

Dental calcification				
Composition		**Shape**		
Dentinal	**Homogenous spherulites**			
Non dentinal	**Lamellar spherulites**	**Amorphous spherulites**	**Irregular**	**Granular**

6.7 The structure of calcifications in relation to age group

True denticles - they occur at early age, the non-dentinal calcifications - they occur in the middle or older age.

Dentinal calcifications

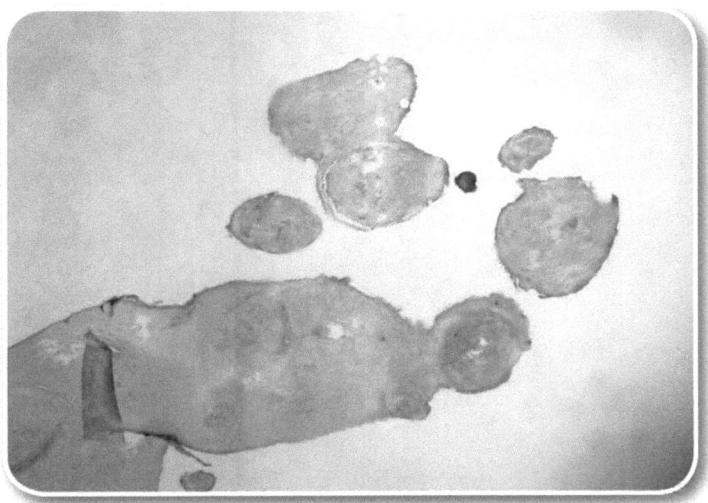

Figure 1.　　HE staining (magnify.10x4), formations of decalcified spherical pulp stones, dentinal composition

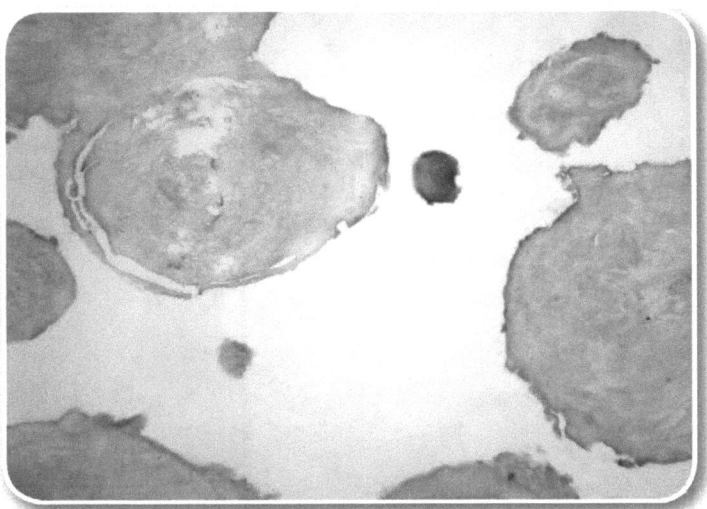

Figure 2.　　HE staining (magnify.10x10), formations of decalcified spherical pulp stones, dentinal composition

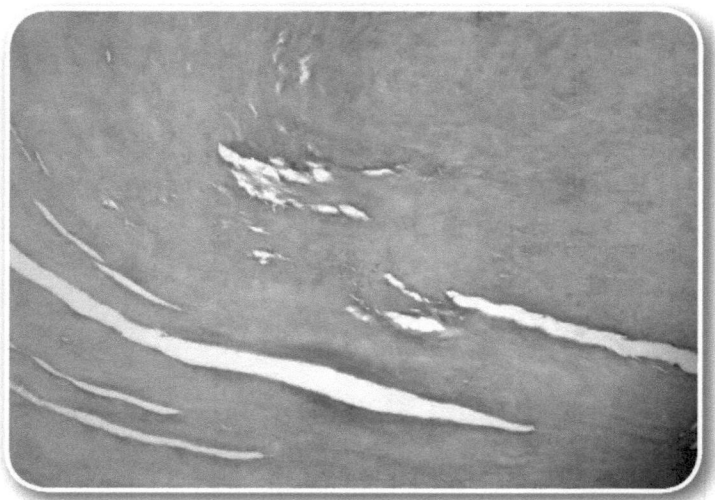

Figure 3.   HE staining (magnify.10x20), formation of decalcified spherical pulp stones, dentinal composition

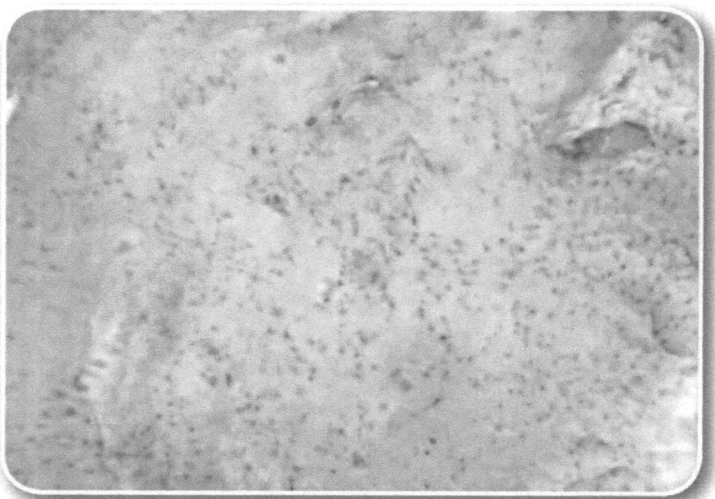

Figure 4.   HE staining (magnify.10x40), formation of decalcified pulp stones, dentinal composition, anarchic dentinal tubules

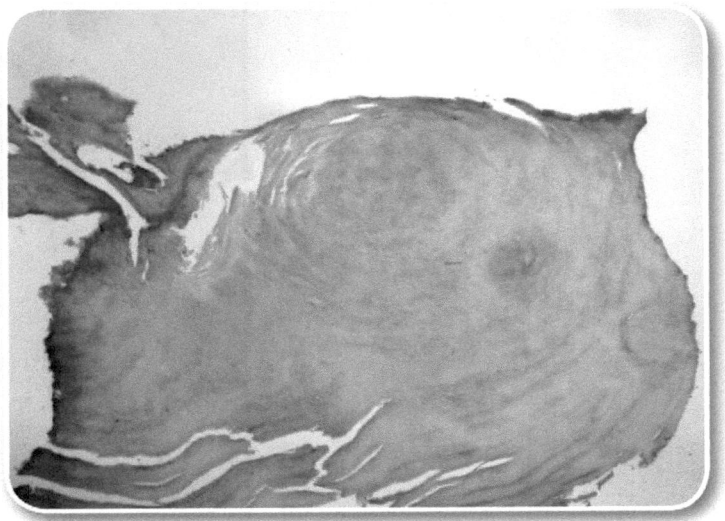

Figure 5. HE staining (magnify.10x4), formation of decalcified spherical pulp stones, dentinal composition

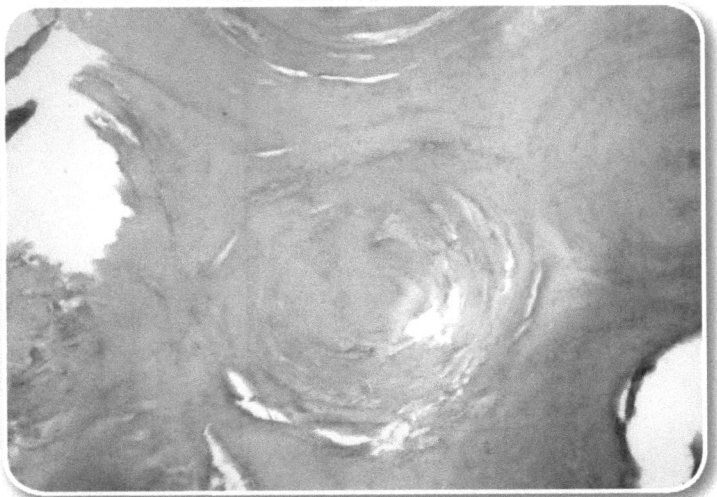

Figure 6. HE staining (magnify.10x10), formations of decalcified spherical pulp stones, dentinal composition, dentinal tubules itself partially with radial disposition, partially with anarchic disposition

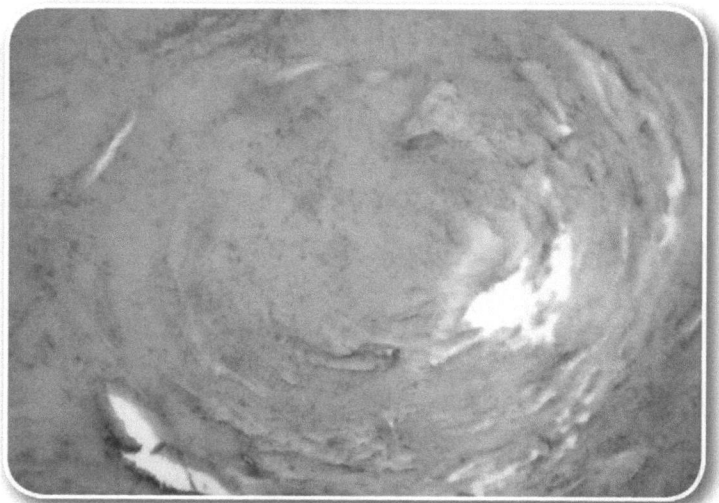

Figure 7.   HE staining (magnify.10x20), formations of decalcified spherical pulp stones, dentinal composition, dentinal tubules itself partially with radial disposition, partially with anarchic disposition

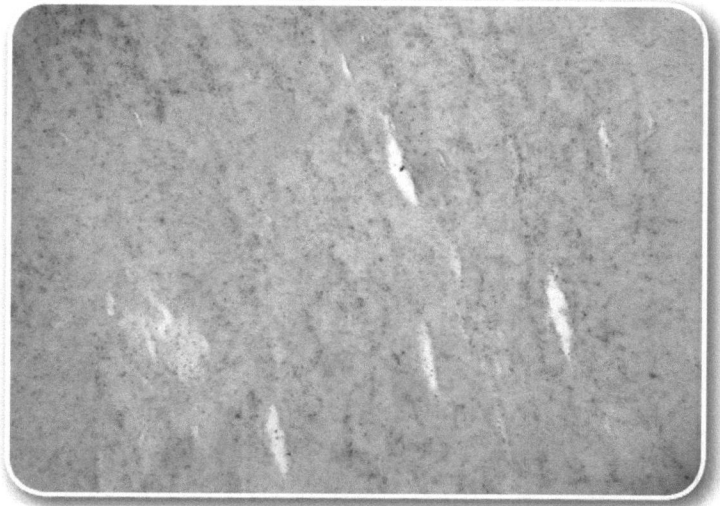

Figure 8.   Von Kossa staining (magnify.10x40), formation of decalcified pulp stones, in organic matrix with punctiform encrustations from calcium

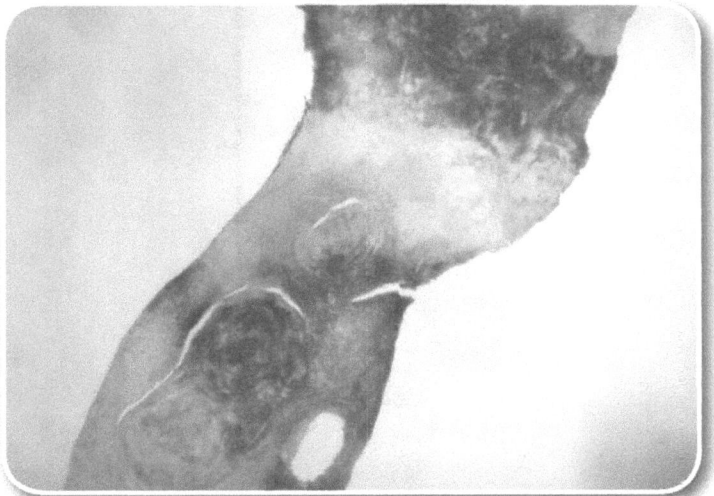

Figure 9.   Masson's trichrome stain (magnify.10x4), figure of visualization of predentin and dentin, predentin coloring green, mature dentin coloring red

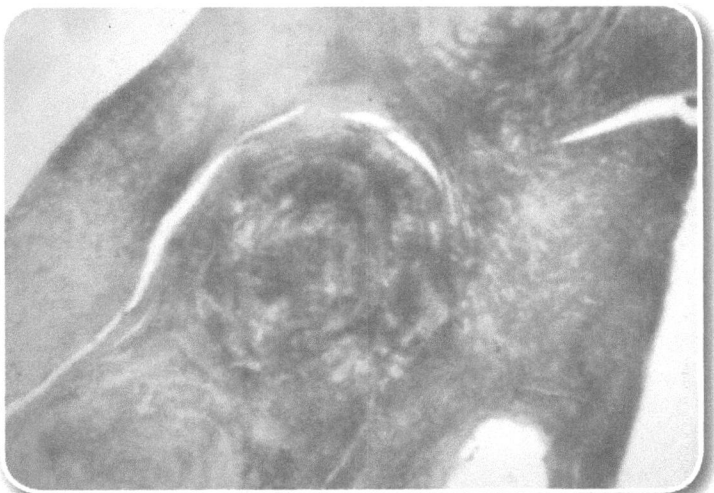

Figure 10.   Masson's trichrome stain (magnify.10x10), figure of visualization of predentin and dentin, predentin coloring green, mature dentin coloring red

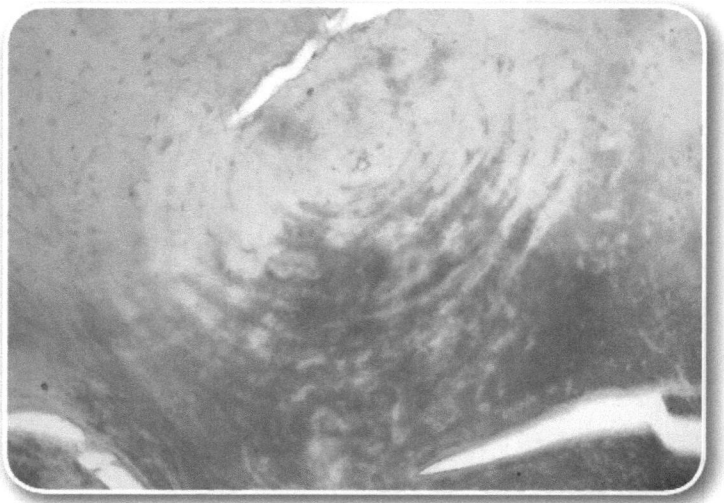

Figure 11.   Masson's trichrome stain (magnify.10x20), figure of visualization of predentin and dentin, predentin coloring green, mature dentin coloring red

Non-dentinal calcifications

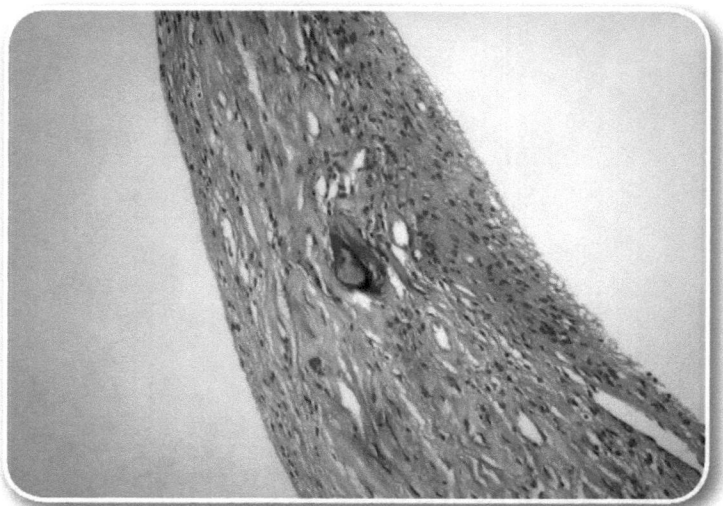

Figure 12.   HE staining (magnify.10x4), formation of solitary partially decalcified pulp stones, oval shape, non-dentinal composition with amorphous compact morphology. Pulp is with reduce cells and hyalinizing connective tissue without inflammation process

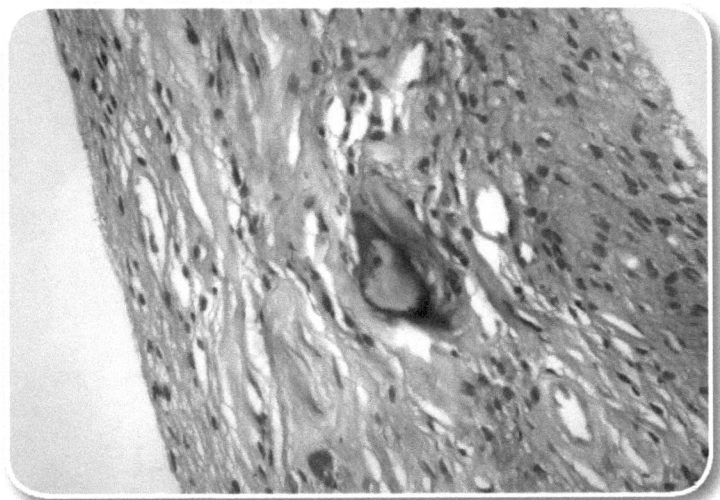

Figure 13. HE staining (magnify.10x20), formation of solitary partially decalcified pulp stones, oval shape, non-dentinal composition with amorphous compact morphology. Pulp is with reducing cells and hyalinizing connective tissue without inflammation process. Down and little left from calculus degenerating sheaf from nerve fibers

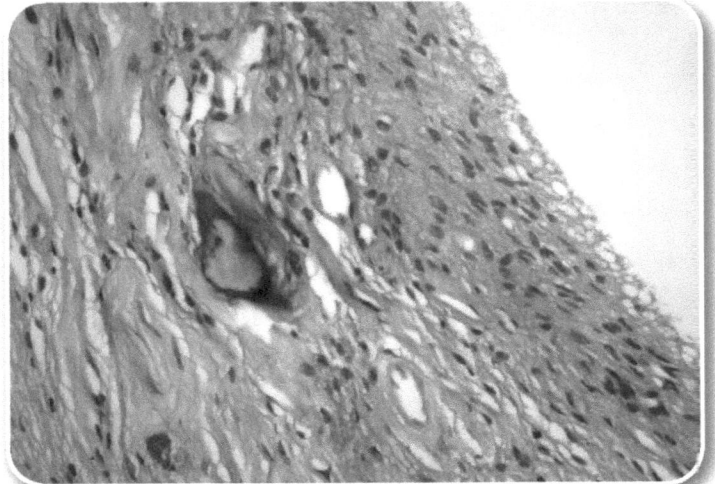

Figure 14. HE staining (magnify.10x25), formation of solitary partially decalcified pulp stones, oval shape, non-dentinal composition with amorph compact morphology. Pulp is with reducing cells and hyalinizing connective tissue without inflammation process. Down and little left from calculus degenerating sheaf from nerve fibers

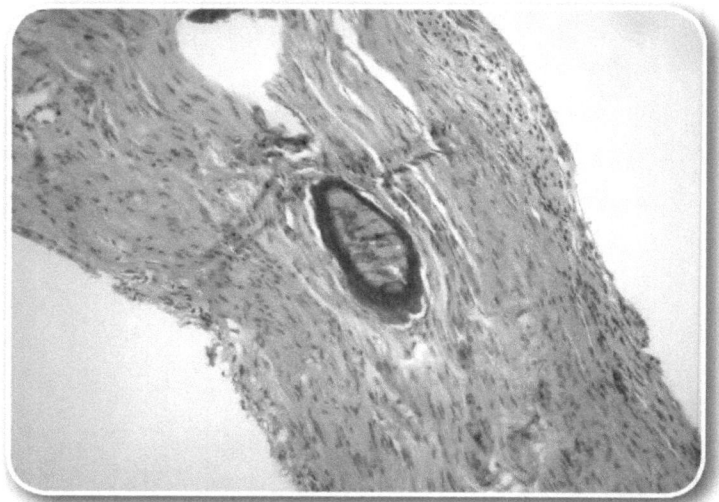

Figure 15.   HE staining, (magnify. 10 x 10), formation of solitary partial decalcinated pulp
stone, oval shape, non-dentinal composition, the structure being partially
lamellar partially compact. In the surrounding there is present hyalinized pulp
stroma with reduction of the vascular compartment

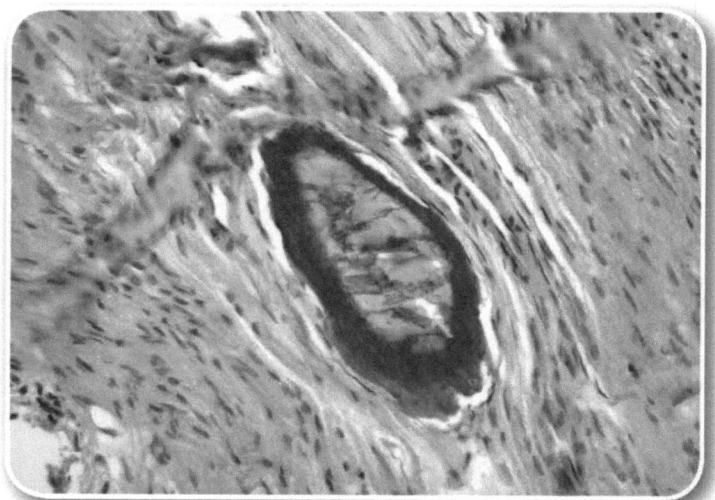

Figure 16.   HE staining, (magnify. 10 x 10), absence of odontoblasts and dentinal tubules

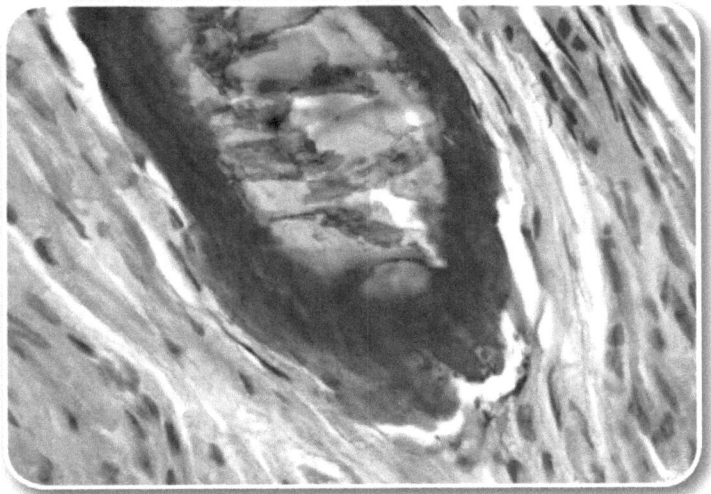

Figure 17. HE staining, (magnify. 10 x 10), the same material of great magnify, details of pulp stone and around storm of pulp

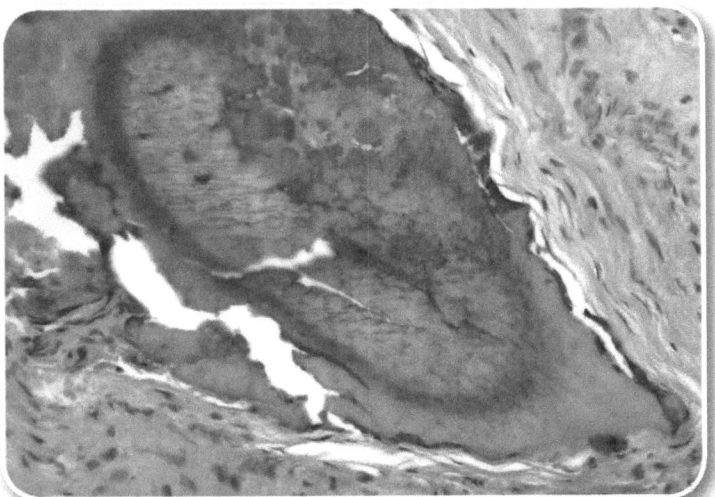

Figure 18. HE staining, (magnify. 10 x 20), formation of solitary pulp stone with composite elements in the structure, towards the periphery with greater dentin content, towards the middle area with transformation of morphology of non-dentin calculus resulting most probably from the abundant deposit of calcium in the organic nidus. Hyalinized pulp in the surrounding area

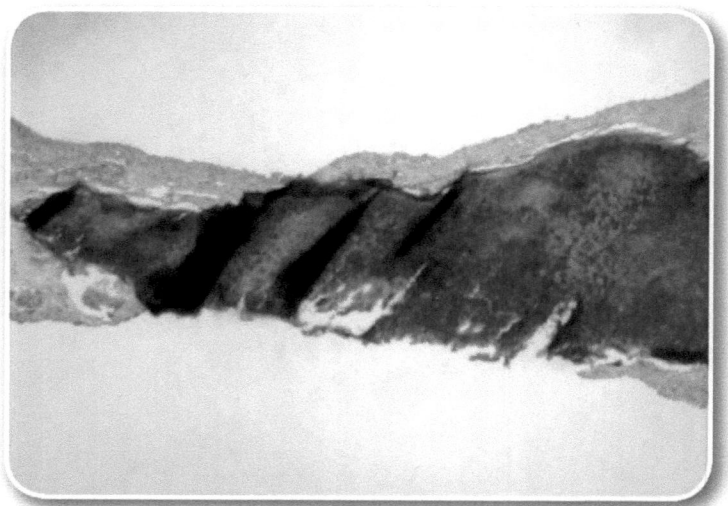

Figure 19.   HE staining, (magnify. 10 x 4), formation of dental calcification, denticle with fine granulated structure, the size of which being such to occupy the pulp almost across all its width and along its length. Visible congested blood vessels

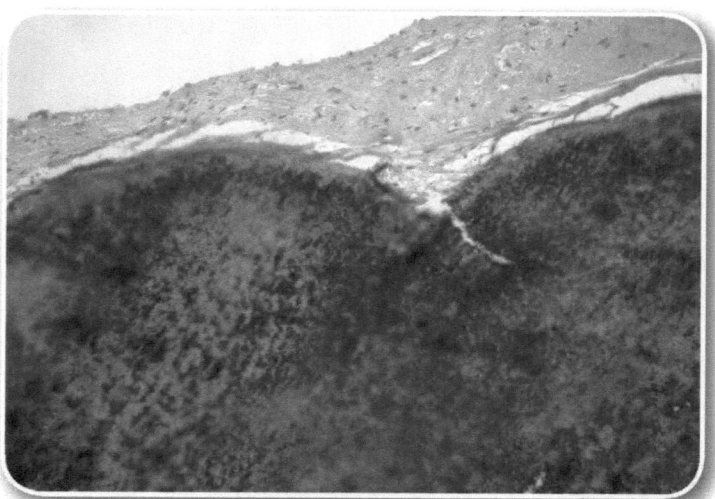

Figure 20.   HE staining, (magnify. 10 x 20), greater zoom than the one of the formation of dental calcification with fine granular structure

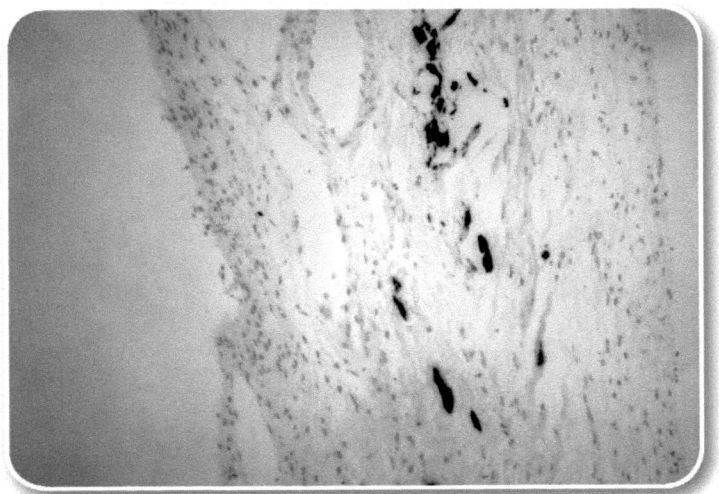

Figure 21.   Von Kossa staining, (magnify. 10 x 10), non-dentinal, more of number, differently of size, partial decalcinated calcifications, known such dystrophic calcification

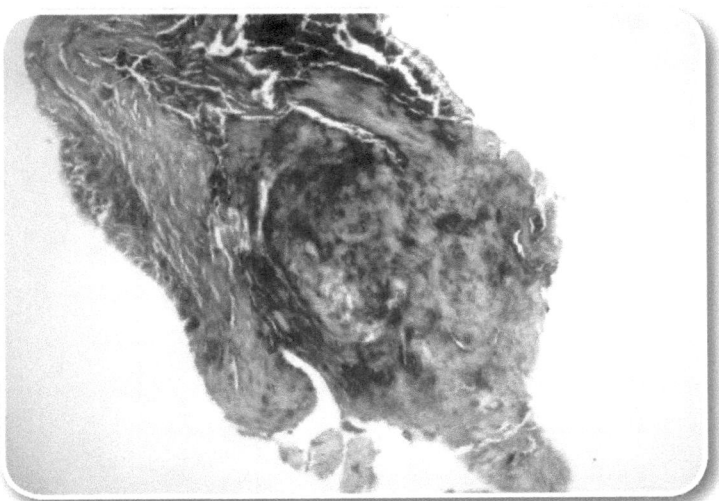

Figure 22.   Gimsa staining, (magnify. 10 x 10), partial decalcinated non-dentinal pulp stone, significant presence of calcium coloring red

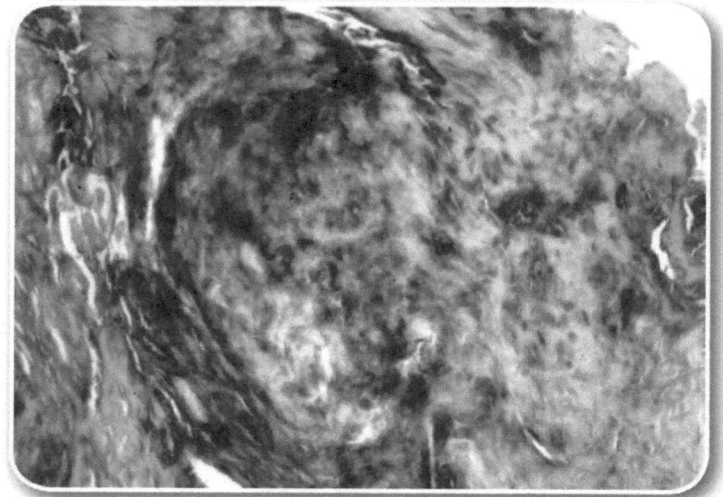

Figure 23.   Gimsa staining, (magnify. 10 x 40), partial decalcinated non-dentinal pulp stone, significant presence of calcium coloring red

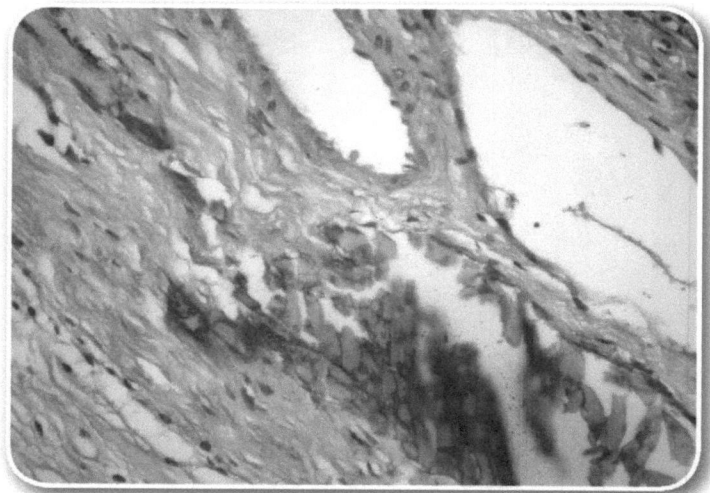

Figure 24.   HE staining, (magnify. 10 x 20), non-dentinal, irregular of shape, amorphous-crystal calcification with neighboring hyalinized pulp and wide free vascular space

7. CLINICAL IMPLICATION

When dental calcifications are classified as non-dentinal, dental practitioner is obligated to send the patient to subsequent or supplementary inspection, primarily ultrasonography survey first to abdomen, for early detecting of calcifications and calculus in other organs.

The practitioners of general medicine and the specialists of nephrology, gastroenterology, cardiology and all other specialties that meet pathologic calcification, physicians who have patients with associate unexplainable long-term headache could refer them to a doctor of stomatology for diagnosis and therapy of possible pulp stone pathology.

8. CONCLUSION

Using the experience from present classifications of dental calcifications and the classifications of other diseases and syndromes, together with this results, can be a reason to propose the following:

1. New classification of dental calcifications, according to the structure:

   • Calcifications with morphological features similar to the structure of dentin,

   • Calcifications with lamellar concentric structure, and

   • Calcifications small granular structure.

2. New classification of dental calcifications, according to their composition:

   • Dentinal and

   • Non-dentinal calcifications, can be confirmed histological.

3. The new classification will enable us to determinate the composition of denticles according to the age of patients, without any histological analysis.

4. When they are classified as non-dentinal, dental practitioner is obligated to send the patient to subsequent or supplementary inspection, primarily ultrasonography survey first to abdomen, for early detecting of calcifications and calculus in other organs.

5. Early detecting of calculi in other organs, can prevent surgery interventions and complications.

9. REASON

As a basis for discussion is the finding that the dental calcifications represent a separate model of pathological calcification, fitting into overall pathological classification, although with different structure and composition.

Literature is rich with descriptions of dental calcifications. The greatest attention is paid to the significance and prevalence of denticles [73,74,75,76,77,78,79]. The influence of the tablet fluoridation on primary teeth is often analyzed [80,81] but studies on the structure of dental calcifications are scarce [80,83] which leaves possibility to try to define it in a more accessible manner, and to clarify this dental entity.

Both from clinical and pathological aspect, it is impossible to avoid the question concerning appropriateness and clarity of terminology that is being actually used. It seems that there is a significant degree of overlapping terms, which impedes notion of dental calcifications and mutual communication. The most frequently used terms such as real denticles, false denticles and dystrophic calcifications, contribute to confusion as do not provide sufficiently precise answer of whether these calculi are calcifications.

What remains untold in huge number of descriptions is the structure of real denticles, which further leaves open the question about what they really are?

Dental calcifications or pulp stones have been extensively studied morphologically.

Structural features of dental calcification, described in our project, showed a morphological picture similar to that of the dentin structure - lamellar, concentric and with fine granular structure. The presented structural features were similar to dentin with smaller quantity of calcium, i.e. predentin, with increased presence of calcium salts in the medium area, which unambiguously shows that there is identical histogenesis of both the dentin and the spherical more or less calcified dental calcifications (Fig.17). This structure of calculi, i.e. calcifications with morphological features of dentin structure, implies that a term "denticle" should be used, although they are also known as "real denticles". Histopathological findings of calcification with lamellar and concentric structure (Fig.15,16 and18) show that there is a rough deposition of calcium salts, absence of fine trabecular-tubular structures, otherwise present in the dental calcification, presence of organic matrix initially, as well as protracted interpolated encrustation with calcium salts. These morphological features allow us to use the term "false denticles", as a part of the wider group of dystrophic calcifications. Therefore this could represent a direction towards a more concrete etiological conditioning of this pathological entity. In our findings, the structure of fine granulated calcifications (Fig.19 and 20) consists of the biggest presence of calcium salts and maximum reduced organic matrix. With reference to the previous 2 groups, this can represent a proof of the time-dimension regarding the dynamics of calcium depositing due to chronic etiological provocation of traumatic or infective origin.

As a separate subgroup in this category also fall the fine granulated multifocal and confluent calcifications along the longitudinal axis of the pulp, dissociated of bundles of hyalinised connecting tissue, rich in collagen. They also get intensively colored with hematoxylin which implies that there is a prevalence of calcium salts compared to the organic matrix.

Being engaged in comparing denticles in the pulp of human teeth and those in cow's teeth, Kodaka et al. [84] emphasize that denticles in the pulp of human teeth contain biological apatite as well as organically dependent and amorphous minerals. According to them, denticles in the pulp of cow's teeth in their medium area contain granulated structures, so called "nidi", which could be thrombi or necrotic blood with erythrocytes. The authors draw a conclusion that such "calcospherulites" in the cow dental pulp are similar to the "spherulitic" dental stones in humans. The human's "nidi" could be present in different parts of the human organism [85]. In the SEM research of various calcified formations of the pulp, Le May and Kaqueler [86] described the presence of resorptive zones at the surface. The authors gave special review on observations of the fractures in the sense of the presence of non-typical organization in places where mineralized masses are compact and homogenous and concentric architecture around the initial central core and linear orientation along the pulp axis, with a display of mineralized fibres and blood vessels [86]. Dard et al [87] assume that there must be extremely important the role of cytoskeleton in the process of imbibing calcification.

The results obtained from the carried out examinations, in our project, showed that dental calcifications, regarding the composition, can be classified such: 1.dentinal [Fig.1-11] and 2. non-dentinal [Fig.12-24] and Table 4. The dentinal calcifications are spherical, nodular, solitary and more numerous, they contain greater amount of organic matrix; they occur at early age and have hamartomatous aspect. The non-dentinal calcifications could be nodular spherical, irregular in shape or with punctform encrustations. They contain smaller amount of organic matrix, they occur in the middle or older age and have inflammatory dystrophic background.

Studies on the composition of dental calcifications are scarce, which leaves possibility to try to define it in a more accessible manner and to clarify this dental entity [51,86]. In a histochemical study of pulpal calcifications, it has been shown that the organic matrix consists of reticular connective tissue fibers and of a ground substance containing glycoprotein's and acid polysaccharides [88]. The mineral phase of pulp calcification has been studied with X-ray energy dispersive spectrometry (EDX) and chemical analysis, and proven that calcium salts are deposited in the form of apatite, possibly carbonate containing apatite [89]. Actually, there is not big difference between the chemical structure of a tooth and denticles

[90]. Bone and tooth formation in the body have similar mechanisms [91] which have many unanswered questions. Apatite formation in the body except in tooth and bone is called pathologic biomineralization, e.g., dental pulp stones, kidney stones, joint calcifications. Interestingly, also environmental apatite stones have almost the same chemical composition as in bone and dentine [92]. The results, obtained from the patient questionnaire, showing high incidence of kidney stones and gall stones in both patients and their parents [92]. Pulp stone can be a predictive marker for kidney stone [93].

We assume that this significant difference is of vital importance since, when a dentist detects and diagnoses a denticle in the coronary part of the pulp, i.e. at the canals' entrance, he/she should immediately send the patient for an ultrasound diagnosis of the abdomen, primarily of the kidneys and the bile. In the majority of our patients a positive diagnosis was established; calculi detected for the first time in the kidneys and/or bile, and often in other organs as well [94].

Pulp stones have been compared to kidney and gall bladder stones (Martin 2002), [95].

The characteristics of the disease, the incidence of new registered cases, the frequency of patients with recidive calculosis, the disease period length and the consecutive organ and organism repercussions, include the pathologic calcification in the group of illnesses with strong social impact.

REFERENCES

1. Boskey AL. Current concepts of the physiology and biochemistry of calcification. Clin Orthop Relat Res.1981;(157):225-57.

2. Anderson HC. Calcific diseases. A concept. Arch Pathol Lab Med.1983; 107970: 341-8.

3. Garimella R., Bi X. Anderson HC., Camacho NP. Nature of phosphate substrate as a major determinant of mineral type formed in matrix vesicle-mediated in vitro mineralization: An FTIR imaging study. Bone. 2006; 38(6): 811-7.

4. Anderson HC. Molecular biology of matrix vesicles. 1:Clin Orthop Relat Res. 1995; (314): 266-80.

5. Anderson HC. Mechanism of pathologic calcification. Rheum Dis Clin North Am. 1988; 14(2): 303-19.

6. Boskey Al. Mineral-matrix interactions in bone and cartilage.1:Clin Orthop Relat Res. 1992; (281): 244-74.

7. Anderson HC. Normal and abnormal mineralization in mammals.1:Trans Am Soc Artif Intern Organs. 1981; 27: 702-8.

8. Boskey AL., Boyan BD., Schwartz Z. Matrix vesicles promote mineralization in a gelatin gel. Calcif Tissue Int. 1997; 60(3): 309-15.

9. Douglas Mulhall and Katja Hansen. Extracted from the book "The Calcium Bomb", 2005.

10. Rushton MA. A case of dentinal dysplasia. Guy's Hosp Rep. 1939;89:369–73.

11. Wang W., Kirsch T. Retinoic acid stimulates annexin-mediated growth plate chondrocyte mineralization.

12. N.R. Kaipatur, M.Murshed, M.D.McKee. Matrix Gla Protein Inhibition of Tooth Mineralization. Journal of Dental Research – J Dent Res, vol. 87, no. 9, pp. 839-844, 2008.

13. Harsha Vardhna Talla, Nandra Kumar Kommineni, Samatha Yalamancheli, Jogendra Sai Sankar Avula and Deepa Chillakuru. A study on pulp stones in a group of the population in Andhra Pradesh, India:An institutional study.J Conserv Dent. 2014; 17(2): 111–114.

14. Sandeep Kumar Bains, Archana Bhatia, Harkanwal Preet Singh, Swati Swagatika Biswal, Shashi Kanth and Srinivas Nalla.Prevalence of coronal pulp stones and its relation with systemic disorders in northern Indian Central Punjabi Population.ISRN Dentistry Volume 2014(2014), Article ID 617590, 5 pages.

15. Aleksova Pavlina, Dental calcifications-reason for special analysis. Masters Degree Paper (MD Paper), 2006.

16. Stenvik A, Mjör IA. Epithelial remnants and denticle formation in the human dental pulp. Acta Odontol Scand. 1970;28:72–8.

17. Moss-Salentijn L, Klyvert MH. Epithelially induced denticles in the pulps of recently erupted, noncarious human premolars. J Endod. 1983;9:554–60.

18. Hillmann G., Geurtsen W. Light-microscopical investigation of the distribution of extracellular matrix molecules and calcifications in human dental pulps of various ages. Cell Tissue Res. 1997;289:145-54.

19. Sundell JR., Stanley HR., White CL. The relationship of coronal pulp stone formation to experimental operative procedures. Oral Surg Oral Med Oral Pathol. 1968;25:579–89.

20. S. Ranjitkar, J. A. Taylor, and G. C. Townsend, "A radiographic assessment of the prevalence of pulp stones in Australians," Australian Dental Journal, vol. 47, no. 1, pp. 36–40, 2002.

21. E.-A. Holtgrave, W. Hopfenmüller, and S. Ammar, "Abnormal pulp calcification in primary molars after fluoride supplementation," Journal of Dentistry for Children, vol. 69, no. 2, pp. 201–206, 2002.

22. O. Bauss, D. Neter, and A. Rahman, "Prevalence of pulp calcifications in patients with Marfan syndrome," Oral Surgery, Oral Medicine, Oral Pathology, Oral Radiology and Endodontology, vol. 106, no. 6, pp. e56–e61, 2008.

23. N. Çiftçioglu, V. Çiftçioglu, H. Vali, E. Turcott, and E. O. Kajander, "Sedimentary rocks in our mouth: dental pulp stones made by nanobacteria," in Instruments, Methods, and Missions for Astrobiology, vol. 3441 of Proceedings of SPIE, pp. 130–137, July 1998.

24. Zeng JF., Zhang W., Jiang HW., Ling LO. Isolation, cultivation and initial identification of Nanobacteria from dental pulp stone.1: Zhonghua Kou Qiang Yi Xue Za Zhi. 2006; 41(8):498-501.

25. Kajander E.O., Çiftçioglu, N., Bjound M. Mineralization by nanobacteria. Proc. SPIE. 1998; 344: 86-94.

26. Kajander E.O., Çiftçioglu N. Nanobacteria: An alternative mechanism for pathogenic intra- and extracellular calcification and stone formation. Proc. Natl. Acad. Sci. USA. 1998; 95: 8274-8279.

27. Neva Çiftçioğlu and David S McKay. Pathological Calcification and Replicating Calcifying-Nanoparticles: General Approach and Correlation. Pediatric Research (2010) 67, 490–499; doi:10.1203/PDR.0b013e3181d476ce.

28. Tadic D, Peters F, Epple M 2002 Continuous synthesis of amorphous carbonated apatites. Biomaterials 23:2553–2559.

29. Zaidi AN, Ceneviva GD, Phipps LM, Dettorre MD, Mart CR, Thomas NJ 2005 Myocardial calcification caused by secondary hyperparathyroidism due to dietary deficiency of calcium and vitamin D. Pediatr Cardiol 26:460–463

30. Carson DA 1998; An infectious origin of extraskeletal calcification. Proc Natl Acad Sci USA 95:7846–7847.

31. Pachman LM, Boskey AL 2006 Clinical manifestations and pathogenesis of hydroxyapatite crystal deposition in juvenile dermatomyositis. Curr Rheumatol Rep 8:236–243.

32. Mc Carty DJ 2008 Basic Ca phosphate and calcium oxalate crystal deposition diseases. In: Porter RS, Kaplan JL (eds) The Merck Manual Online. Merck & Co., Inc., Whitehouse Station. Accessed at December 5, 2009

33. Kajander EO, Çiftçioglu N 1998 Nanobacteria: An alternative mechanism for pathogenic intra- and extracellular calcification and stone formation.Proc Natl Acad Sci USA 95:8274–8279.

34. Puskás LG, Tiszlavicz L, Rázga Z, Torday LL, Krenács T, Papp JG 2005 Detection of nanobacteria-like particles in human atherosclerotic plaques.Acta Biol Hung 56:233–245.

35. Miller VM, Rodgers G, Charlesworth JA, Kirkland B, Severson SR, Rasmussen TE, Yagubyan M, Rodgers JC, Cockerill FR III, Folk RL, Rzewuska-Lech E, Kumar V, Farell-Baril G, Lieske JC 2004 Evidence of nanobacterial-like structures in calcified human arteries and cardiac valves. Am J Physiol Heart Circ Physiol 287:H1115–H1124.

36. Çiftçioğlu N, McKay DS, Kajander EO 2003 Association between nanobacteria and periodontal disease. Circulation 108:e58–e59.

37. Çiftçioglu N, Björklund M, Kuorikoski K, Bergström K, Kajander EO 1999 Nanobacteria: an infectious cause for kidney stone formation. Kidney Int56:1893–1898.

38. Pavlina Aleksova. Nanobacteria – CNPs the possibility of bacterial association of the dental calcifications. International Journal of Science and Research (IJSR). ISSN (Online) Volume 4,issue 4, 2015. Page 7: 3173-3175.

39. Pavlina Aleksova. Nanobacteria can be reason for creating sialoliths. International Journal of Science and Research (IJSR). ISSN (Online): 2319-7064. Volume 4,issue 3, 2015. Page 5: 2248-2250.

40. Pavlina Aleksova, Daniela Velevska-Stefkovska. Calcifying nanoparticles (CNPs) in human gallstones. International Journal os Science and Research (IJSR). ISSN (Online): 2319-7064. Volume 3,Issue 12, 2014. Page 3.

41. Aleksova Pavlina. Nanobacteria – CNPs the possibility of bacterial association of the dental calcifications in correlation with the salivary gland stones. International Journal of Science and Research (IJSR). ISSN (Online): 2319-7064.Volume 4,issue 4, 2015. Page 7: 3176-3178.

42. Kim JW, Simmer JP. Hereditary dentin defects. J Dent Res. 2007;86:392–9.

43. Ballschmiede G. Dissertation, Berlin, 1920. Quoted. In: Herbst E, Apffelstaedt M, editors. Malformations of the Jaws and Teeth. New York: Oxford University Press; 1930.

44. Rushton MA. A case of dentinal dysplasia. Guy's Hosp Rep. 1939;89:369–73.

45. Witkop CJ., Jr Hereditary defects of dentin. Dent Clin North Am. 1975;19:25.

46. Sangamesh G. Fulari and Deepti P. Tambake. Rootless tetth: Dentin dysplasia type I. Contemp Clin Dent. 2013 Oct-Dec; 4(4): 520–522.

47. Plačková A., Vahl J. Ultrastructure of Mineralizations in the Human Pulp. Caries Res 1974; 8:172-180. (DOI:10.1159/000260105).

48. Johnson and G. Bevelander. Histogenesis and Histochemistry of Pulpal Calcification. DENT RES October 1956 35: 714-722.

49. Moss-Salentijn L, Hendricks- Klyvert M. Calcified structures in human dental pulps. Journal of Endodontics 14(4):184-189, 1988.

50. Appleton J, Williams MJ (1973) Ultrastructural observations on the calcification of human dental pulp. Calcified Tissue Research 11, 222–37.

51. Goga R, Chandler NP, Oginni AO. Pulp stones: a review. International Endodontic Journal, 41, 457–468, 2008.

52. Irvin Glickman B.S., D.M.D., Gerald Shklar, B.Sc., D.D.S.,M.S. The effect of systemic disturbances on the pulp of experimental animals. Oral Surgery, Oral Medicine, Oral Pathology. Vol. 7, Issue 5; Pages: 550-558.

53. Parekh S, Kyriazidou A, Bloch-Zupan A, Roberts G. Multiple pulp stones and shortened roots of unknown etiology. Oral Surg. Oral Med. Oral Pathol. Oral Radiol Endod. 2006; 101(6): e 139-42.

54. Kantaputra PN, Sumitsawan Y, Schutte BC, Tochareontanaphol C. Van der Woude syndrome with sensorineural hearing loss, large craniofacial sinuses, dental pulp stones, and minor limb anomalies: Report of a four-generation Thai family. Am J Med Genet.2002;108:275–80.

55. I.A. Mjor and J.J. Pindborg. Histology of the Human Tooth. Munskgaard Copenhagen, 1st edition, 1973.

56. Baume LJ. The biology of pulp and dentine.A historic, terminologictaxonomic, histologic-biochemical, embryonic and clinical survey.Monographsin oral science. Vol. 8. Basel: S Karger, 1980:174-8.

57. Miller WA. Pulp calcifications in a taurodont tooth. Br Dent J 1969;126:456-9.

58. Weinreb M, Michaeli Y. Possible mechanisms of induction of dentinogenesis. Med Hypotheses 1984;13:163-9.

59. Bernice Thomas, ManojChandak, Adityavardhan Patidar, Bharat Deosarkar, Harshit Kothari. Calcified Canals – A Review. Journal of Dental and Medical Sciences (IOSR-JDMS) e-ISSN: 2279-0853, p-ISSN: 2279-0861.Volume 13, Issue 5 Ver. IV. (May. 2014), PP 38-43.

60. Willman W. Numerical incidence of calcification in human pulps [Abstract]. J Dent Res 1934;1:160-1.

61. Bab I, Lustmann J, Azaz B, Gazit D, Garfunkel A. Calcification of noncollagenous matrix in human gingiva: a light and electron microscopic study. JOral Pathol 1985; 14:573-80.

62. Harrop JT, Mackay B. Electron microscopic observations on healing dental pulp in the rat. Arch Oral Bio11968;13:365-85.

63. Aoba T, Ebisu S, Yagi T. A study of the mineral phase of pulp calcification. J Oral Patho11980;9:129-36.

64. CL.Udove and MA Sede. Prevalence and Analysis of Factors Related to Ooccurrence of Pulp Stone in Adult Restorative Patients. Ann Med Health Sci Res. 2011 Jan-Jun; 1(1): 9–14.

65. Hakan Çolak, Ahmed Arif Çelebi, M. Mustafa Hamidi, Yusuf Bayraktar, Tuğba Çolak and Recep Uzgur. Assessment of the Prevalence of Pulp Stones in a Sample of Turkish Central Anatolian Population. The Scientific World Journal Volume 2012 (2012), Article ID 804278, 7 pages.

66. R. Kronfeld and P. E. Boyle, Histopathology of The Teeth and Their Surrounding Structures, Henry Kimpton, London, UK, 4th edition, 1955.

67. A. Arys, C. Philippart, and N. Dourov, "Microradiography and light microscopy of mineralization in the pulp of undemineralized human primary molars," Journal of Oral Pathology and Medicine, vol. 22, no. 2, pp. 49–53, 1993.

68. Sreeelakshmi, Tejavathi Naqaraj, Pooja Sinha, Rahul Dev Goswami, Bhavana Thymagondalu Veerabasaviah. A radiographic assessment of the prevalence of idiopathic pulp calcifications in permanent teeth: A retrospective radiographic study. Journal of Indian Academy of Oral Medicine & Radiology. 2014, Volume : 26, Issue 3; Page: 248-252.

69. Mahajan P., Monga P., Bahunguna N., Bajaj N. Principles of management of calcified canals. Indian J Dent Sci 2010;2(Suppl):3-5.

70. Stella A, Sisco RG, Hernandez E, Osorio S, Di Piramo S. Contribucion al estudio de lasformacionescalcicas del organopulpar y periodontal. Origen, evotucion y significacionclinica. An FacOdontol 1966;12:55-68.

71. Fridrichovsky H. ZurHistologie der Dentikel. Z Stomato11927;25:124- 57.

72. Orban B. Epithelial rests in the teeth and their supporting structures. Proc Am Assoc Dent Schools 1929;121:133.

73. Baghadi SV, Ghose JL, Nahoom YH. Prevalence of pulp stones in a teenage Iragi group. J Endodon, 1988; 14:309- 311.

74. Delivanis HP, Sauer GJ. Incidence of canal calcification in the orthodontic patient. Am J Orthod, 1982; 82:58-61.

75. Hamasha al-Hadi A, Darwazeh A. Prevalence of pulp stones in Jordanian adults. Oral Radiol Endod, 1998; 86:730-732.

76. Lin CT, Roan RT, Rou WJ, Chen JH, Chuang FH, Hsieh TY. A radiographic Assessment of the Prevalence of Pulp Stones in Taiwanese. Svenska Massa, 2003; 11:12-15.

77. Olivares HML, Ovalle CJM. Prevalence of pulp stones. Rev ADM, 2001; 58(4):130-137.

78. Pavlina Aleksova. A Radiographic Assessment of the Prevalence of Pulp stones in Premolars Regarding the Dental Arches. International Journal of Science and Research (IJSR) ISSN (Online): 2319-7064.

79. Stajer AL, Kokai LE. Incidence and origin of dental pulp stones. Fogorv Sz, 1997; 90:119-123.

80. Holtgrave EA, Hopfemüler W, Ammar S. Tablet fluoridation influences the calcification of primary tooth pulp. J Orofac Orthop, 2001; 62:22-35.

81. Holtgrave EA, Hopfenmüler W, Ammar S. Abnormal pulp calcification in primary molars after fluoride supplementation. J Dent Chil, 2002; 69:201-206.

82. Hussein I, Uthman AA. An unusual calcification of the pulp: A case report. J Endodon, 1982; 8:33-34.

83. Nakagawa K, Yoshida T, Asai Y. Ultrastructure of initial calcification on exposed human pulp applied with autogenons dentin fragments. Bull Tokyo Dent Coll, 1981; 30:137-143.

84. Kodaka T, Hiroyama A, Mori R, Sano T. Spherulitic brushite stones in the dental pulp of a cow. Journal of Electron Microscopy, 1998; 47:57-65.

85. Kumar S, Chadra S, Jaiswai JN. Pulp calcifications in primary teeth. J Pedod, 1990; 16:218-220.

86. Le May O, Kaqueler JC. Scanning electron microscopic study of pulp stones in human permanent teeth. Scaning Microsc, 1991; 5:257-267.

87. Dard M, Kerebel B, Orly, Kerebel LM. Transmission electron microscopy of the morphological relationship between fibroblast and pulp calcification in temporary teeth. J Oral Pathol, 1988; 17:124-128.

88. Le May O, Kaqueler JC. Electron probe micro-analysis of human dental pulp stones. Scanning Microsc. 1993 Mar; 7(1):267-71;discussion 271-2.

89. T, Aoba, S. Ebisu, and T. Yagi, "A study of the mineral phase of pulp calcification", J. Oral. Pathol 9 pp 129-136, 1980. 8

90. J. L. Rabinowitz, E. Korostoff, D. W. Cohen, and S. Orlean, "Varitaions in dental calculi composition and structure", J. Dent. Res. 48, pp. 1216-1218, 1969.

91. H. C. Hodge, and L. S, Wah, "Calculus formation", J. Periodont. 21, pp. 211-221, 1950.

92. Neva Ciftcioglu, Vefa Ciftcioglu , Hojatollah Vali , Eduardo Turcott and E. Olavi Kajander. Sedimentary rocks in our mouth: Dental pulp stones made by Nanobacteria.

93. De la Garza RV, Tamez de Villarreal A. Possible relationship of urinarylithiasis and some oral disorders. ADM. 1976;33:49–52.

94. Pavlina Aleksova, Vladimir Serafimoski, Mira Popovska, Milčo Ristovski. Pulp stones can help in detection of calculus in the kidneys and/or in the bile–fact or fiction? CONTRIBUTIONS. Sec. Med. Sci., XXXIV 2, 2013.

95. Martin AP. A radiographic assessment of the prevalence of pulp stones. Aust Dent J. 2002 Dec;47(4):355-6; author reply 356.

96. Qualtrough AJ, Mannocci F. Endodontics and the older patient. Dent Update 2011;38:559-62.

97. Pavlina Aleksova. Calcifications in the tooth pulp. Book, National and university library "Ss. Climent Ohridski", Skopje, 2012. ISBN 978-608-65454-0-6.

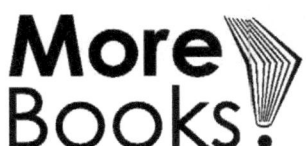
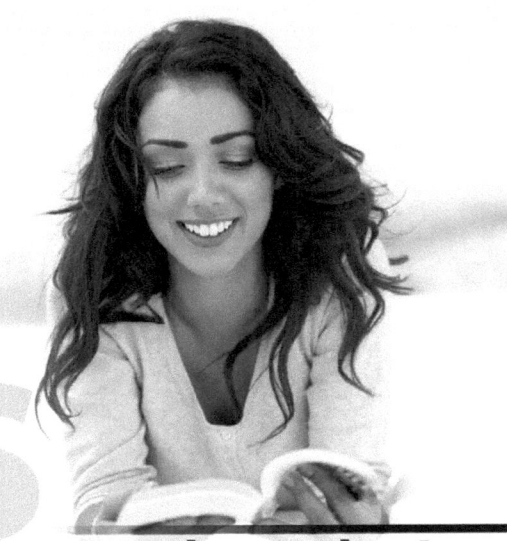
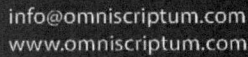
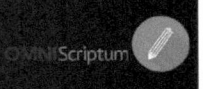

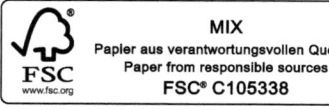